INSTRUCTOR'S MANUAL TO ACCOMPANY
KINESIOLOGY

MOVEMENT IN THE CONTEXT OF **ACTIVITY**

DAVID PAUL GREENE, PhD, MS, OTR

Associate Professor
Department of Occupational Therapy
Colorado State University
Fort Collins, Colorado

With illustrations by
David Paul Greene, PhD, MS, OTR,
and Avtar Dunaway, OTR

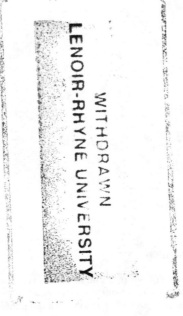
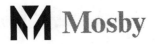 Mosby

St. Louis Baltimore Boston Carlsbad Chicago Minneapolis New York Philadelphia Portland
London Milan Sydney Tokyo Toronto

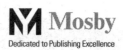

Mosby
Dedicated to Publishing Excellence

A Times Mirror
Company

Publisher: John Schrefer
Executive Editor: Martha Sasser
Senior Developmental Editor: Amy Christopher
Project Manager: Gayle May Morris
Associate Production Editor: Lisa M. Kearney
Designer: Renée Duenow
Manufacturing Manager: David Graybill

Cover Photo © PhotoDisc, Inc.

Composition by Top Graphics
Printing/binding by Plus Communications

Mosby, Inc.
11830 Westline Industrial Drive
St. Louis, Missouri 63146

International Standard Book Number 1-556-64477-9

99 00 01 02 03/9 8 7 6 5 4 3 2 1

Preface

This instructor's manual has been written to provide suggestions for instructors. The intention is to stimulate ideas for teaching, not limit them. Many who teach from this text will have numerous educational strategies and ideas of their own. In cases where instructors have less experience from which to draw, these ideas are offered as a starting point. Also to this end, transparency masters of some of the more helpful figures in the text have been included at the end of this manual. These pages have been perforated and can easily be removed for use.

Each of the chapters from the text is represented with a chapter outline, summary, learning objectives, laboratory activities, multiple-choice exam questions (with answers in bold font), and transparency masters. Both the learning objectives and the laboratory activities are written for student readers. The laboratory activities have additional comments to instructors that relate to suggestions for emphasis in teaching. These same activities, without comments, have been included in the text appendices for easy reference by students as a laboratory manual.

In general, instructors vary in their opinions as to whether students should be given test questions ahead of time to structure their preparation for exams. The multiple choice exam questions listed for each chapter have been generated largely from the learning objectives provided in this manual. The same learning objectives have been included in the text appendices as a study guide for students. Instructors who prefer short answer and essay test formats will find the objectives may be used as discussion or essay questions.

David Paul Greene

Contents

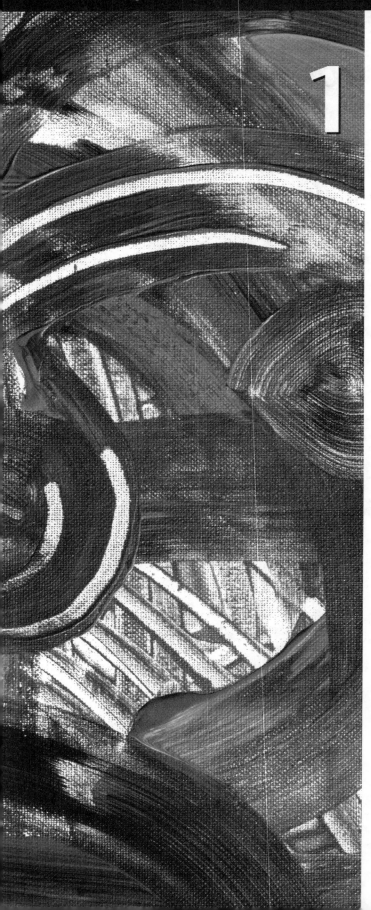

1

Biomechanics, Kinesiology, and Occupational Therapy

A Good Fit

CHAPTER **OUTLINE**

BELIEFS AND DEFINITIONS

MECHANISTIC AND TRANSFORMATIVE PHILOSOPHIES

A BIOMECHANICAL FRAME OF REFERENCE
Limitations of Biomechanical Approaches

INTEGRATION OF BIOMECHANICS WITH MODELS OF PRACTICE

SUMMARY

CHAPTER **SUMMARY**

Kinesiology *is the study* of movement from the perspective of three physical sciences: musculoskeletal anatomy, neuromuscular physiology, and biomechanics. The complexity of these three fields of study often makes their introduction into activity analysis an exercise in examining the "trees that make up a forest." Occupational therapy (OT) practitioners must recognize that kinesiology provides a limited perspective or point of view. Focusing on a specific movement or adaptation must be done with recognition of the larger, real-life environment and the individual's role.

It is important to examine kinesiology and the biomechanical frame of reference in comparison to other frames of reference and models used in the profession as well as occupational therapy's philosophical base. Through awareness of the breadth of the practice, kinesiology may be better used to improve musculoskeletal function in order to contribute to a functional occupational role. Improved musculoskeletal function isolated from the occupational contexts of self-care, work, and play has no place in OT practice.

Learning Objectives

- Define *kinesiology* and identify the three physical sciences that contribute to it.
- Describe why kinesiology is considered a narrow approach to movement.
- Identify the basic belief on which OT practice is based.
- Identify the factors influencing individual performance that become clear when movement is viewed within the context of activity.
- Briefly describe and differentiate mechanistic and transformative philosophies.
- Briefly describe and differentiate the reconstructive, orthopedic, and kinetic models of practice.
- Describe the value of the rehabilitation model as a guide to kinesiologic thinking.

Laboratory Activities

Interview faculty members to determine the philosophy of the department and the models on which the departmental curriculum is based. (*Comment: It may be helpful to lead students to the department's most recent accreditation file for clearly documented information on models and frames of reference pertinent to the department.*)

Exam Questions

1. Kinesiology is the study of movement from the perspective of
   a. Anatomy, physiology, and biology
   b. Anatomy, physiology, and biomechanics
   c. Physiology, physics, and mechanics
   d. Anatomy and physiology

2. Movement should be studied and understood
   a. Strictly in an anatomical context
   b. With emphasis on joint motion for motion's sake
   c. In the context of real life environments
   d. Only in a biomechanical context

3. The ultimate value of intervention based on kinesiology is
   a. The correctness of the biomechanics
   b. The degree that it facilitates adaptive process for an individual
   c. The amount of joint range restored
   d. The restored ability of the individual to perform repetitions of movement against resistance

4. A view of the body as a machine whose inner working parts are independent of the mind is consistent with
   a. Mechanistic philosophy
   b. Transformative philosophy
   c. An open systems model
   d. b and c

5. Models of OT practice that are accustomed to the transformative philosophy include those of
   a. Ayres and King
   b. Reilly and Kielhofner
   c. Baldwin and Taylor
   d. Licht and Dunton
   e. a and b

6. Using a kinesiologic approach within the rehabilitation model
   a. Makes rehabilitation more mechanistic
   b. Broadens the application of kinesiology
   c. Ensures attention to adaptation, not just remediation
   d. b and c

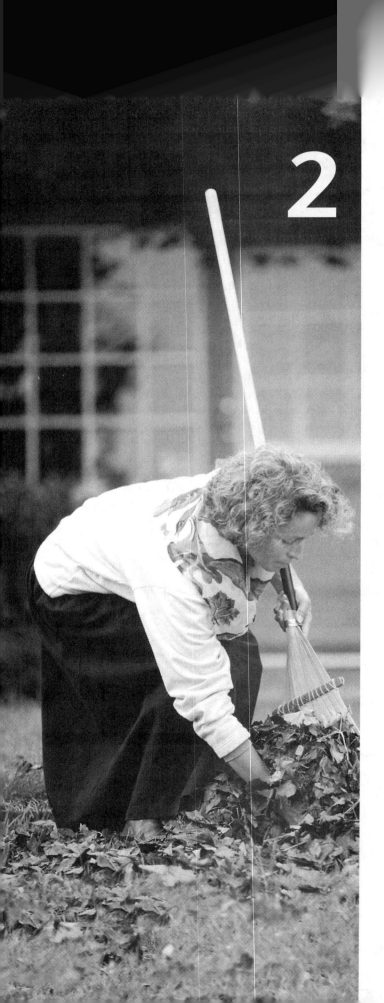

2 The Study of Human Movement

Concepts from Related Fields

CHAPTER SUMMARY

Occupational therapy practitioners need to be familiar with concepts of medicine and physics in order to understand and apply principles of biomechanics and kinesiology to functional activity. The vocabulary and concepts outlined in this chapter are a part of every problem presented in the chapters that follow. Most OT students feel comfortable with the concepts of medicine, but for many, physics will be a strange territory. The concepts of physics should become more friendly as we move through the text and apply them to human activity.

Learning Objectives

- Describe the major skeletal movements in terms of planes (surfaces on which the movements occur) and axes (around which the movements are centered).
- Demonstrate the three types of muscle contraction and describe how the two muscle attachments move in each.
- Define *excursion* and describe its effect on muscle length.
- Differentiate the agonist, antagonist, and synergist in a description of muscle action.
- Demonstrate correct use of the terms used to communicate various muscle grades (words and numbers).
- Describe the use of a goniometer to measure joint range of motion and differentiate active and passive joint ranges of motion.
- Provide one-line definitions of the various italicized terms under "Medical Diagnoses Affecting Movement."
- Differentiate scalar and vector quantities in terms of their measurements.
- Differentiate mass and weight, and identify which of the two also is described as force.
- Describe normal force and compare it with shear force.

Laboratory Activities

Identify various forces at work around the room. Identify three different forces by considering the following common activities:

1. The resistance encountered when you move objects by sliding them along the floor
2. The force involved when you pull up the window shades
3. The force that makes you tired at the end of the day
   (**Comment:** *These three forces are friction, muscular force, and gravity, respectively. Students may identify the force involved in pulling up the window shade as gravity, since the shade does have weight. Although this is correct, try to lead them to think about the internal force, muscular force, used in overcoming the weight of the shade.*)

Exam Questions

1. Sagittal plane movements of the wrist occur around
   a. Front-to-back axes
   b. Side-to-side axes
   c. Front-to-back axes

2. The strength test usually performed *first* in MMT is the test for
   a. Poor strength
   b. Normal strength
   c. 3/5 strength
   d. Good strength

3. Considering two biceps muscles, one from a very tall person with long extremities and the other from a smaller person with short extremities, which biceps has greater (longer) excursion?
   a. The one from the tall person since that biceps is longer
   b. The one from the smaller person since that biceps is shorter
   c. They are the same since both are biceps muscles
   d. Whichever biceps has the greater cross section also will have the greater (longer) excursion

4. An extension *movement* against resistance (as in pushing someone away) requires
   a. Concentric contraction of the flexors
   b. Concentric contraction of the extensors
   c. Eccentric contraction of the extensors
   d. Isometric contraction of the extensors

5. When a muscle *concentrically contracts*, it gets
   a. Longer
   b. Shorter
   c. Stronger
   d. Weaker

6. A quantity that can be measured only at a specific moment in time because it implies movement is a
   a. Scalar quantity
   b. Vector quantity

7. The muscle that works opposite a muscle responsible for a specific movement is the
   a. Agonist
   b. Synergist
   c. Antagonist

8. The difference between weight and mass is that
   a. Weight is mass as affected by gravity's pull
   b. Mass is weight as affected by gravity's pull
   c. Weight is a scalar quantity
   d. Mass is a vector quantity

9. Osteoporosis, osteogenesis imperfecta, and avascular necrosis all are diagnoses affecting
   a. Muscle
   b. Tendon
   c. Bone
   d. Skin

10. Tensile and compressive forces are examples of
    a. Normal forces
    b. Shear forces
    c. Friction
    d. Stress

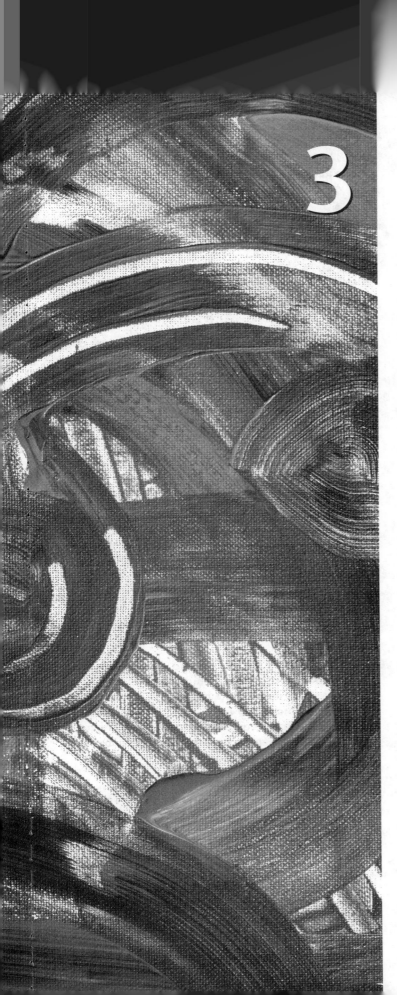

Gravity

A Constant Force

CHAPTER **SUMMARY**

Newton *envisioned the force* of gravitational attraction as something similar to the attraction of magnets. Einstein envisioned space as a fabric where large objects, such as planets, stars, and black holes, created deep pockets that drew smaller objects, such as light rays, inward on a curved trajectory. The conceptual models of these two great mathematicians have kept physicists employed for centuries.

For our purposes, the specific details of the conceptual models are less relevant. In the realm of practical application on earth, objects are pulled downward to the earth in direct proportion to their mass. Although the force of that attraction depends on mass, the acceleration of all objects is constant, and a larger, heavier object will fall to the ground just as fast as a smaller, lighter one. The larger, heavier object will require more force to push it over the edge than the smaller, lighter one. We use these important concepts to visualize gravity's effect on movement, by drawing objects complete with vectors that demonstrate gravity's ever-present influence.

Learning Objectives

- Describe one way in which gravity influences motor development.
- Demonstrate how the center of gravity is approximated.

- Perform the brief calculations and measurements necessary in the identification of an object's center of gravity.
- Determine the center of gravity of the entire body based on the segmental centers of gravity.
- Convert an object's mass (in kilograms) to its weight (in newtons), illustrating how mass is converted to force through the multiplication of mass by the constant for the acceleration of gravity.

Laboratory Activities

Identify various movements of the human musculoskeletal system and the positions this system holds that are caused by the force of gravity. (**Comment:** *This is a good time to encourage differentiation between the movement used to get into a position and the position itself. This differentiation will be important later as students learn formal biomechanical analysis.*)

- ○ In the upright (standing) position, begin with a flexed shoulder, elbow, and wrist and hold the position. Next, relax one joint at a time, starting proximally and ending with the wrist. List each motion and position caused by gravity in the standing position. What movement does gravity cause at each joint in this standing position? Which joint positions are held by gravity? (**Comment:** *Students should observe that gravity extends the shoulder, elbow, and wrist and holds these positions. Ensure that they start in the position as directed and encourage them to move slowly, one joint at a time.*)
- ○ In the supine position on a mat, leave the shoulder extended and flex the elbow slightly past 90 degrees. Next, allow the elbow to move by relaxing all muscle contractions. What is gravity's effect? (**Comment:** *In this position, gravity should be seen to hold the shoulder extended, flexing the elbow. It would hyperextend the shoulder if there was not the support of the mat. Gravity's effect depends on the position of the body.*)

Exam Questions

1. The center of gravity of a uniform object is located
   a. Toward one end of the object
   b. At the center of the object
   c. Outside of the object

2. The location of the center of gravity of a person is affected by
   a. The position of the body
   b. The positions of the various segments
   c. The constant for the acceleration of gravity
   d. a and b
   e. All of the above

3. A wristband weight labeled 5 kg actually weighs
   a. 5 kilograms
   b. 50 newtons
   c. 50 pounds
   d. 5 pounds

4. The location of the center of gravity of a wheel is
   a. Outside the wheel
   b. Throughout the circumference of the outer edge of the wheel
   c. Toward the bottom of the wheel
   d. Dependent on the speed the wheel spins

5. Compared with the standing position, the location of a person's center of gravity within the body while seated in a wheelchair is
   a. Lower
   b. Higher and more posterior
   c. Higher and more anterior
   d. No different

6. How would standing on the right lower extremity to reach into a cabinet affect the body's center of gravity?
   a. It would move it to the right.
   b. It would move it lower.
   c. There would be no effect on the location of the center of gravity.

7. How would reaching upward into a cabinet affect the center of gravity of the reaching forearm?
   a. It would move it to the right.
   b. It would move it lower.
   c. The forearm's center of gravity would move upward with the forearm, but would not change in its location within the forearm.

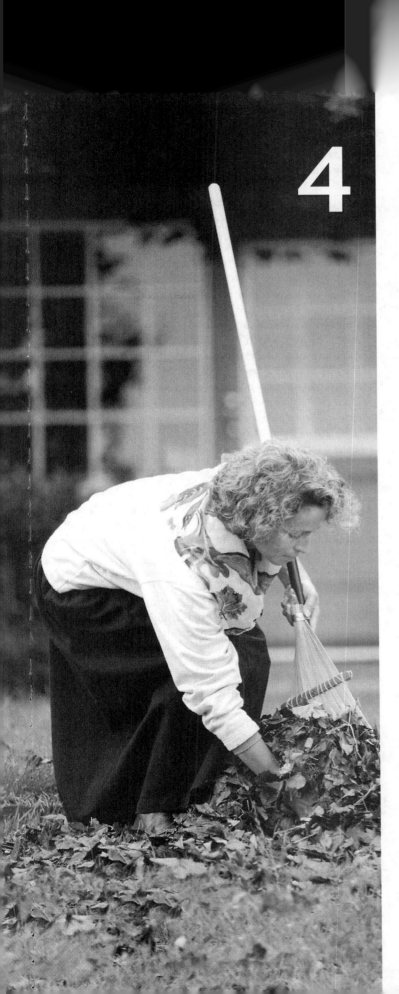

4

Linear Force and Motion

CHAPTER **OUTLINE**

CHAPTER **SUMMARY**

The topics in this chapter all point to the need for OT practitioners to understand their observations of functional activity. When we fail to understand what we see, we simply turn to other sources for ideas to solve our problems. We match our observation to a problem on a list and use the solution suggested by that particular protocol. This "cookbook" approach limits therapy to (1) finding a problem on a list, (2) using other people's solutions for problems, and (3) settling for a solution that does not exactly match all the unique aspects of an individual's life. Each observation represents a separate, novel situation, and a few fundamental laws can explain many different problems. As we develop a greater sense of how these laws interconnect, our understanding of what we observe deepens and our solutions become more effective.

Learning Objectives

- Provide examples of each of Newton's three laws.
- Describe the conditions of force equilibrium when an individual is seated (at rest) in a chair.
- Demonstrate the three types of muscle contraction and describe the movements of the two muscle attachments in each.
- Define the effect of excursion on muscle strength in a concentric contraction.
- Describe what is meant by excursion requirements of movement at a joint.
- Describe what happens to a muscle when its antagonistic motion occurs.
- Describe the change in distance between the origin and insertion of a muscle in a concentric contraction and how this differs from that in an eccentric contraction.
- Describe what happens to the origin and insertion of a flexor muscle when the joint is pulled into extension by an outside force.
- Identify and briefly describe each example of each type of external force described in the chapter.
- Define and differentiate *force magnitude, force orientation,* and *internal (muscular) force direction.*
- Differentiate the determinants of muscular force and excursion.
- Explain how forces are combined through addition and subtraction to determine the resultant force in a tug-of-war game.
- Explain both the parallelogram and polygon methods for the combination of multiple forces when two individuals push a cart.

Laboratory Activities

- As in the activities in Chapter 2, identify various forces at work around the room. Consider a typical window shade with a drawstring in terms of equilibrium of forces. When the shade is pulled up and stays up, is this equilibrium? If so, how is it established? What are the forces involved? (**Comment:** *The equilibrium of up and down forces involves the force of friction in the locking mechanism holding the drawstring balanced by the downward force of gravity on the shade.*)
- Compare the excursion of a long spring with a short one. Also compare the force of recoil of one bungee cord with the force of four identical bungee cords pulled simultaneously. Draw parallels to relationships between normal muscle excursion and force capability. (**Comment:** *The longer spring, representing the longer muscle, has a greater excursion. A single bungee cord compared with four bungee cords represents a muscle with a small*

cross section compared to one with a larger cross section. The four together are thicker and provide more resistance to stretch than the one alone, similar to the muscle with the greater bulk that is capable of a larger force of contraction.)

- Identify examples of force equilibrium around the room (for example, sitting in a chair or on the mat).
- Working with a partner, hook a bungee cord to the doorknob of a closed door and stretch the cord by backing from the door one or two steps. Instruct someone to turn the knob to allow the door to swing open. The same person should hold onto the door to allow it to swing only as far as the bungee shortens. Measure the distance the door travels when the bungee recoils and the distance through which the bungee contracts. Repeat this action but stand farther from the door the next time. What is the name of the distance through which the bungee contracts? What does the movement of the door represent? (**Comment:** *Identify this distance of contraction as the excursion; the door movement represents the active range of motion of the joint. Point out that the bungee contracts for every bit that the door opens. Opening the door wider requires more excursion. The same is true for muscles and joints.*)

Exam Questions

1. What is insufficient in the active contraction of multijoint muscles, preventing them from producing full, simultaneous motion in all of the joints they cross?
   a. Excursion
   b. Passive stretch

2. What is the situation called (as described above) in which a muscle contracts but is unable to cause complete movement in all of the joints it crosses?
   a. Passive insufficiency
   b. Active insufficiency

3. Passive insufficiency involves a multijoint muscle having inadequate
   a. Distal excursion
   b. Proximal excursion

4. When a muscle contracts, the muscle and tendon exhibit
   a. Active, distal excursion
   b. Passive, distal excursion
   c. Active, proximal excursion
   d. Passive, proximal excursion

5. If an extensor tendon is unable to fully glide distally in its path because it is bound up in scar tissue,
   a. **Flexion, the antagonistic motion, will be limited**
   b. Extension will be affected, but flexion will be unimpaired

6. Considering two biceps muscles, one from a very tall person with long extremities and the other from a smaller person with short extremities, which biceps has greater (longer) excursion?
   a. Whichever biceps has the greater cross section also will have the greater (longer) excursion
   b. **Whichever biceps has the longer resting length**

7. One muscle is stronger than another depending on which has the greatest
   a. Active excursion
   b. Passive excursion
   c. **Cross section (area)**

8. Joint position at the beginning of a muscle contraction
   a. Affects only muscle excursion necessary for the movement
   b. **Affects muscle excursion and strength**
   (HINT: *Consider beginning the contraction of the biceps in a position near full elbow flexion.*)

9. The absolute maximum strength capacity of a muscle depends on
   a. **The muscle's cross section (area)—the larger, the stronger**
   b. The muscle's resting length—the longer, the stronger

10. An extension *movement* (as in slowly letting down a heavy object) requires
    a. Concentric contraction of the flexors
    b. Concentric contraction of the extensors
    c. Eccentric contraction of the extensors
    d. **Eccentric contraction of the flexors**
    e. b and d

11. When the long finger flexors (flexor digitorum profundus) contract (concentric) flexing the finger,
    a. The tendon of the long flexor exhibits excursion proximally
    b. The tendon of the long extensor exhibits excursion distally
    c. Both flexor and extensor tendons go through active excursion in the proximal direction
    d. There is excursion only in the flexor tendon, and it is passive and distally directed
    e. **a and b**

12. The flexor digitorum profundus (long flexor of the fingers) is in *active* insufficiency
    a. When the wrist and fingers are simultaneously extended
    b. When there has been a maximum of passive/distal excursion
    c. When this muscle is passively stretched across all of its joints simultaneously
    d. **When this muscle has exhausted its active excursion**

13. If the long finger extensors contract in a concentric contraction and extend the wrist *before* fully extending the fingers,
    a. **The extensors will run out of excursion and be unable to completely extend the fingers**
    b. The extensors will exhibit passive insufficiency
    c. Complete finger extension will occur—it will just take longer

14. When a muscle concentrically contracts, it gets _____ and at its extreme it will be capable of _____ force.
    a. Longer; greater
    b. Shorter; greater
    c. **Shorter; less**
    d. Longer; less

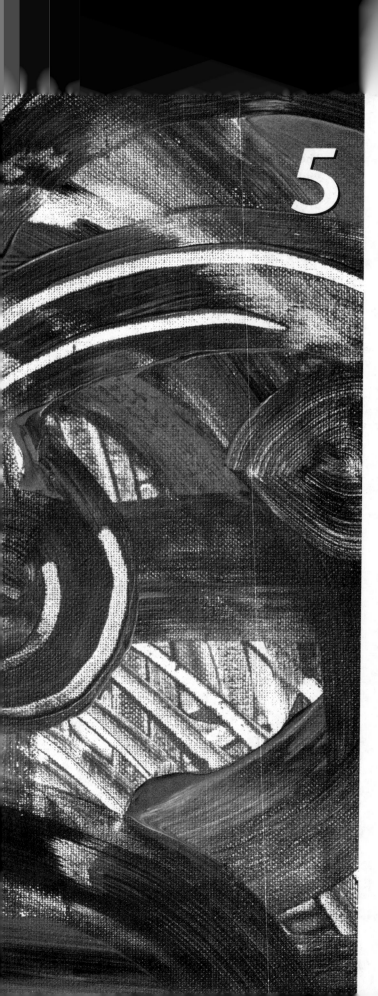

5

Rotary Force, Torque, and Motion

CHAPTER **OUTLINE**

ROTARY MOTION

TENDENCY TO ROTATE

EQUILIBRIUM OF TORQUES

LEVER SYSTEMS
Everyday Levers
Musculoskeletal Levers

EXTERNAL AND INTERNAL TORQUE
Torque Value
Changing Factors During Constant Torque

SUMMARY

CHAPTER **SUMMARY**

W*e are accustomed to associating* force with movement and more force with faster movement or greater strength. Rotary movement expands our thinking and leads us to realize that there is more to consider than simply amount of force. The placement of force with respect to the axis of motion also is important. The two together, magnitude and placement, result in a tendency to set bony segments and external objects into motion in a circular path. Circular motions and the tendencies of different muscles to cause them will consume much of our attention in adapting for difficult movements.

Learning Objectives

- Differentiate rotary and linear motion based on (1) the velocity of points in a bar moving in a line versus in a circle and (2) the orientation of the bar.
- Describe the difference in the effect of the amount of force used in linear versus rotary motion.

- Provide a synonym for the term torque.
- Identify factors used in the determination of linear and rotary equilibrium.
- Identify the angle of pull at which all the muscle's force is used for the rotary movement of the joint.
- Identify the angle of pull at which the moment arm is the longest.
- Identify at which moment arm the movement is strongest.
- Provide everyday examples of each lever system.
- Explain why most musculoskeletal levers are class III levers.
- Explain how changing the force's angle of pull and the muscle length affect the tendency of the force to rotate the lever at the joint.
- Identify the lever and axis of various musculoskeletal segments.

Laboratory Activities

- In small groups discuss why each of the following statements actually says the same thing about the strongest movement of the musculoskeletal segment:
  - Elbow flexion is strongest when the joint is flexed to 90 degrees because the flexors pull from their best angles and the muscle length is good.
  - The torque produced by the elbow flexors is greatest at 90 degrees of flexion because the moment arm is at its longest length and the actin and myosin overlap is ideal for force production by the muscle fibers. (*Comment: 1. Saying a motion is "strongest" is the lay equivalent of greatest "torque produced." 2. A moment arm improves—is longer—as the "angle of pull" away from the segment increases, up to 90 degrees. This angle of pull is between the force vector and the segment it pulls into motion. 3. The best muscle length for producing strength is at a point where the actin and myosin overlap is optimal.*)
  - The torque produced by the elbow flexors is greatest at 90 degrees of flexion because the force of flexion is farthest from the axis (has the greatest perpendicular distance) and the actin and myosin overlap is optimal for force production. (*Comment: Saying the "force of flexion is farthest away from the axis" is synonymous with saying "the moment arm is at its longest length"; this occurs when the angle of pull of the force is at its best—90 degrees.*)
- Working in pairs, use a dynamometer to generate your own isometric torque curve. Set it on the second grip-span setting and attempt three grip efforts, measuring grip strength at 40 degrees of wrist extension, neutral position, and full wrist flexion. For each effort, plot the force of grasp on one axis and the wrist position on the other, using axis labeling as in the following illustration.

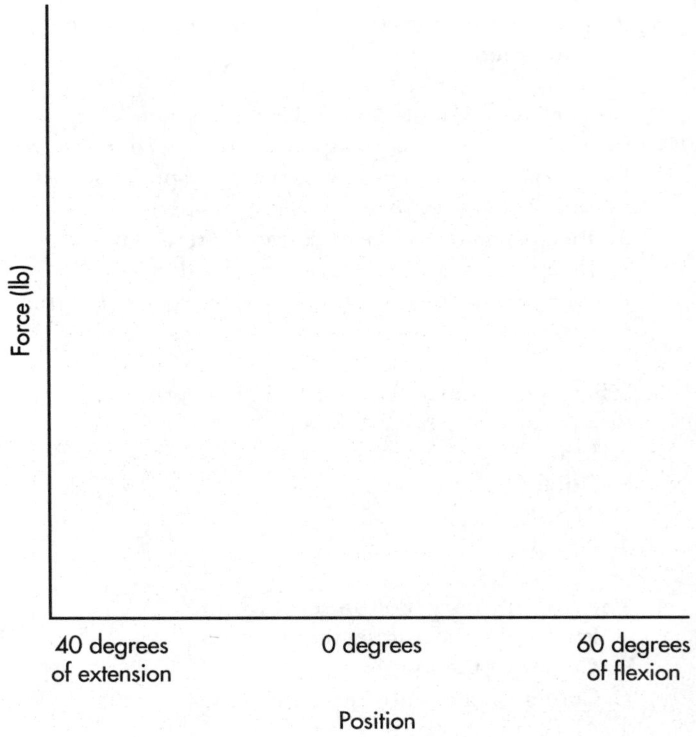

Force (lb) [vertical axis]

| 40 degrees of extension | 0 degrees | 60 degrees of flexion |

Position

Discuss the following points related to the graph:
- What happens to the strength of the grasp as the wrist position changes? (*Comment: Strength should be greatest with 40 degrees of wrist extension. Make sure that the students hold the three desired positions. They tend to go into wrist extension with grasp even though they think they are performing grip in neutral and 60 degrees of flexion.*)
- Identify the specific effect on the finger flexors when the grip begins from different wrist positions. (*Comment: The main concept here is that the long finger flexors are shorter at the beginning of grip in each position other than wrist extension. Being shorter, myofilament overlap is not as good for force production as when the wrist is extended. The flexors are closer to active insufficiency as wrist flexion increases simultaneously with grip [finger flexion].*)

Exam Questions

1. Why is there greater ability of a muscle group to produce a movement at a specific point in the range, as shown on an isometric torque curve?
   a. Moment arm increases combined with a psychological effect
   b. Increased moment arm and more favorable muscle length
   c. Requirement for distal excursion changes with movement
   d. Movement brings the active group closer to active insufficiency

2. In repetitive elbow flexion and extension as performed in eating (or slurping) soup, does the insertion of the biceps move faster or slower than the spoon held in the hand? Do they move at the same speed?
   a. Biceps insertion moves slower than the spoon
   b. Biceps insertion moves faster than the spoon
   c. Biceps insertion and the spoon move at the same speed

3. What type of motion is described in the previous question considering the elbow and the shoulder?
   a. Linear
   b. Rotary
   c. Tensile
   d. Normal

4. The axis in rotary motion serves as the
   a. End of the moving segment
   b. Center of the motion
   c. Center of each moving segment
   d. All of the above

5. You are trying to flex your elbow against the resistance created by a weight held in the hand. The elbow will flex if
   a. The force of the biceps is greater than the force of the resistance
   b. The torque toward flexion produced by the force of contraction of the biceps is greater than the torque toward extension
   c. The effort begins with the elbow in a middle position of 90 degrees of flexion

6. Torque is described as the
   a. Tendency of a force to cause rotation
   b. Tendency of a force to cause either rotary or linear motion
   c. Force of rotation (*HINT: Is torque dependent only on force?*)
   d. a and b

7. If you are holding a 20-pound weight in your hand with your elbow flexed to 90 degrees (middle position), what do you know about the force of the elbow flexors?
   a. They are contracting in an isometric contraction
   b. As a group they are producing 20 pounds of force toward flexion to balance the 20 pounds of extension force produced by the weight
   c. As a group they are contracting with far greater than 20 pounds toward flexion
   d. The flexion tendency (created by flexors) is equal to the extension tendency (created by weight)
   e. c and d

8. As the elbow joint moves *from beginning to middle position,* the movement of the insertion of the biceps in an arc around the axis results in
   a. The muscle force pulling at a greater distance from the axis—an increasing moment arm
   b. Maintenance of the distance between the force and the axis—an unchanging moment arm

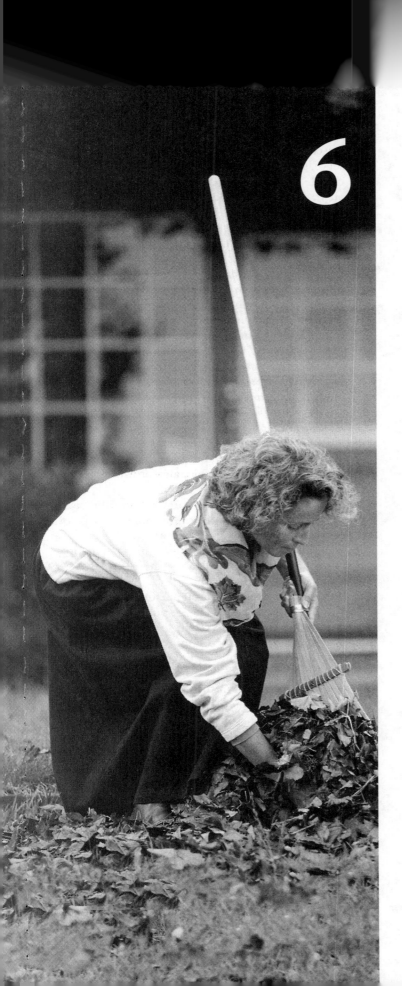

6 The Head and Torso

CHAPTER **SUMMARY**

The bony and soft tissue structures of the head, neck, and trunk provide a stable but flexible shell to protect vital organs, a stable base for movement of the extremities, and a moving contribution to extend upper extremity reach. In spite of its remarkable design, the back was never meant to lift even the weight of the trunk itself. The vertebral extensors, with their short moment arms, produce more compression than extension force. Maintaining upright posture requires little extensor force and causes minimal compression of the intervertebral disks. In contrast, lifting with the back uses a great deal of extensor force and introduces enough compression to damage disks.

Biomechanics can explain and provide solutions for many common problems associated with positioning. Basic principles covered in this chapter should serve as a basis for addressing two of the most common problems an OT practitioner will encounter:

1. Providing external support from the pelvis upward along the vertebral column when internal stability fails as a result of muscle weakness.
2. Assessing restraints from the perspective of positioning principles. Consider failure and discomfort from restraints as a result of poor positioning.

Learning Objectives

- Differentiate between open- and closed-chain hip movements.
- Describe the relationship between lumbar curve and hamstring length.
- Describe the three basic pairs of movements and the nature of vertebral column movement.
- Describe the normal and pathological curves of the vertebral column.
- Explain the effects of unilateral and bilateral contractions of vertebral muscles.
- Explain how movements differ in direction and plane according to the relationship of the force to the axis.
- Describe movements and muscle functions in the trunk that relate to and accompany upper-extremity movements.
- Describe how the trunk remains balanced against the downward pull of gravity.
- Describe the relationship between head and neck position and the force experienced by the cervical intervertebral disks.
- Explain the relationship between rotary force (extension) and compression force during activation of the back extensors.
- Explain the role of pelvic stabilization in seating.
- Describe the basic biomechanics of one common restraint system.

Laboratory Activities

- Draw the muscle masses (not individual portions) of the three erector spinae groups and the transversospinalis group onto a template of the trunk skeleton (see Figure 6-7 in the text), indicating the general direction of the fibers.
- Study your own upper extremity while performing (1) elbow and shoulder flexion to bring food to your mouth (self feeding pattern) and (2) movement in which your hands rest on the front edge of the water

fountain and you lower your head and upper trunk to take a drink:

- ○ Identify the joints and segments that make up the chain.
- ○ Describe the upper-extremity movement you observe, specifically the movement of the end of the chain. Is the movement linear or rotary? (*Comment: The musculoskeletal movements of the upper extremity at each joint are rotary.*)
- ○ Is the movement an example of open- or closed-chain movement? (***Comment:*** *Self-feeding involves open-chain movements. Instruct students to key into the hand, the distal end of the chain, moving freely in space in relation to the trunk. They can watch the insertions of shoulder abductors and flexors and elbow flexors moving instead of the origins. Letting yourself down to the level of the water fountain involves closed-chain motion of the upper extremity. The hands are fixed and not moving while the trunk moves in relation to the hands. For watching origins, make the point that this elbow flexion involves eccentric contractions of triceps, controlling the effect of gravity. Watch the olecranon stay in position and the infraglenoid tubercle [origin of long head of triceps] move toward the olecranon.*)

- Using a skeleton of the trunk with the rod removed so that the curves are flexible, answer the following questions:
- ○ Identify the three normal curves. Describe each curve's location (superior or inferior) and type of convexity (anterior versus posterior).
- ○ Manipulate the pelvis to demonstrate the flattening of the lumbar curve. Which way must the pelvis be tilted to flatten this curve?
- ○ With one person loosely stabilizing the trunk in an upright position, carefully pull on four cords attached to the trunk. Attach three cords posteriorly to the vertebral column to simulate the extensor and the left and right lateral flexor muscle groups of the trunk. Also attach a cord anteriorly to the lower sternum to simulate trunk flexors. Remember that these muscles originate largely from the pelvis. As you pull on the cords to balance or move the column, pull from the origin. Notice the large movement arm for the flexors and the short movement arm for the extensors and lateral flexors.

- Use your own bodies and observe movements in a partner: For each reach, identify (1) elbow and shoulder movements and positions held during the reach, (2) scapular movement and position held during the reach, and (3) trunk movement and position held during the reach:
- ○ Reach forward as far as possible with both arms, putting all your effort into the movement. In other

words, reach with more than arm's length. (*Comment: Observe forward trunk flexion.*)

○ Reach directly to the left or right (again, in an extreme reach). (*Comment: Observe lateral flexion.*)

○ Reach as far as possible with the right arm for an object located in front of and to the left of the left shoulder. (*Comment: Observe trunk rotation—the anterior trunk moves to face the left.*)

Exam Questions

1. Balancing the upper body at the hip against the pull of gravity in bilateral standing,
   a. The hip flexors activate if the center of gravity falls anterior to the side-to-side axis
   b. The hip extensors activate if the center of gravity falls anterior to the side-to-side axis

2. The main effect of the back extensors when trying to "straighten up" from a forward flexed position is to
   a. Extend the vertebral column
   b. Compress the intervertebral disks
   c. Cancel out lateral flexion effects and produce pure extension of the column

3. Contraction of the right transversospinalis muscle
   a. Extends the trunk
   b. Laterally flexes the trunk to the right (same side)
   c. Rotates the trunk anterior to the left
   d. Laterally flexes and extends the trunk to the opposite side
   e. Rotates the trunk anterior to the right

4. The *normal* curves of the vertebral column include
   a. Lumbar curve—convex anterior
   b. Lumbar curve—convex posterior
   c. Thoracic curve—convex to the right
   d. Cervical curve—convex posterior

5. *Bilateral* contractions of the trunk lateral flexors result in
   a. Total lack of motion but good stability of the column
   b. Cancellation of lateral flexion—net effect is extension
   c. Diminished vertebral curves
   d. Extra lateral flexion—all other motions canceled

6. Extreme reach of the right arm across the front to reach an object left of the left shoulder requires
   a. Trunk rotation, anterior to right
   b. Trunk forward flexion
   c. Trunk lateral flexion to the right
   d. Trunk extension
   e. Trunk rotation, anterior to left

7. Leaning to the right requires contraction of which muscle group to balance against gravity?
   a. Trunk flexors
   b. Left trunk lateral flexors
   c. Right and left lateral flexors
   d. Right transversospinalis
   e. Right trunk lateral flexors

8. The sternocleidomastoid muscle
   a. Functions to produce neck extension with "chin tuck"
   b. Flexes the head on the neck
   c. Flexes the head and neck onto the trunk
   d. All of the above

9. Trying to touch the toes with over-shortened hamstrings results in
   a. Too much anterior pelvic tilt and exaggerated lumbar lordosis
   b. Too little closed-chain hip flexion and reverse of lumbar curve

10. Closed-chain motions involve stabilization of the _____ and movement of the _____.
    a. Muscle origin; distal end of the segment
    b. Muscle insertion; distal end of the segment
    c. Distal end of the segment; muscle insertion
    d. Muscle insertion; proximal end of the segment
    e. Muscle origin; muscle insertion

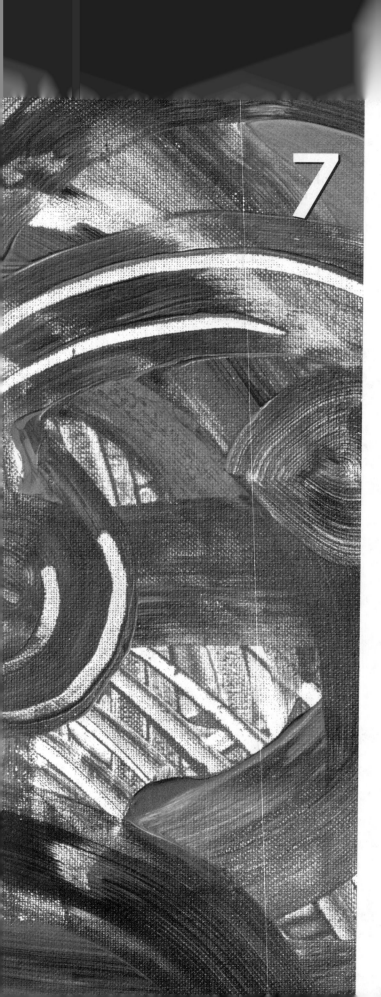

7

The Proximal Upper Extremity

CHAPTER **OUTLINE**

CHAPTER **SUMMARY**

T*he more deeply* we look at the shoulder and elbow, the more interesting we discover they are. Our hands get where we want them to go because of freedom in the sternoclavicular joint and movement of the scapula. The rotator cuff muscles are cuffs but much more than simple rotators. Scapular muscles sometimes move the trunk. Ten-pound handbags can result in joint reaction forces nearing 50 pounds. The elbow flexes and extends sometimes because of muscles that move the shoulder. All these mysteries make perfect sense after we apply a few relatively simple concepts from biomechanics.

Learning Objectives

- Describe the joints of the shoulder complex and the elbow in terms of their classifications and degrees of freedom, including the plane and axis associated with each degree of joint freedom.
- Differentiate scapular from glenohumeral movement.
- State the major movements and movers of the shoulder complex.
- Describe how arrows are used to demonstrate the analysis of muscle forces affecting the shoulder and elbow.
- Describe the scapular movement and stabilization that accompany glenohumeral movement.
- Describe the separate contributions of scapular rotation and glenohumeral abduction to shoulder abduction when an individual raises the hand above the head.
- Explain the main effect of the deltoid compared with that of the supraspinatus in early glenohumeral abduction.
- Explain the biomechanical basis for shoulder subluxation.
- List the various roles of the rotator cuff muscles.
- Describe how manual muscle testing is an example of an isometric torque curve.
- Describe how manual muscle testing is an example of equilibrium of torques.
- Describe how the biceps long head can "become" an abductor of the glenohumeral joint.
- List the combination of joints necessary for flexion and extension and pronation and supination of the forearm.
- Describe how the use of the biceps in elbow flexion can depend on the forearm's position.
- Explain the role of the biceps in supination.
- Describe the contribution of the wrist joint to forearm pronation and supination range of motion.

Laboratory Activities

- To track scapular movement, observe various motions in a partner. Have your partner reach forward as far as possible with one arm, pushing the hand in front of the chest:
  - Identify the scapular motion, using proper terminology. (*Comment: This is a good opportunity for students to closely watch the scapula and understand why the movement is called scapular protraction or scapular abduction, considering the movement of the vertebral border away from the column. Make sure they move in straight protraction and not upward scapular rotation so they can see the pure movement.*)
  - Return your partner to a resting position (seated upright). Palpate your partner's scapular spine, acromion, vertebral scapular border, and inferior scapular angle.
  - Instruct your partner to move again as before and palpate the movement of the scapula, paying close attention to the movement of the vertebral border from the vertebral column. How many centimeters would you estimate the scapula moved?
  - Instruct your partner to return to a resting position and to move through complete abduction, bringing the hand high into the air above the head. Palpate the scapular movement, paying close attention to the inferior angle. How many centimeters did it move? What would you call this scapular motion? (What other terms have you heard used to describe this motion?) (*Comment: This, in contrast to the first movement, should involve upward scapular rotation. The easiest part of the scapula to track is the inferior angle. Make sure students find it at rest and then after the movement. Most students underestimate the amount the inferior angle sweeps laterally and cannot find it well if they did not try to visually track it from the beginning. It is a good time to provide both terms, upward scapular rotation [watching the glenoid] or lateral scapular rotation [watching the inferior angle].*)
- Using the goniometer, measure shoulder abduction to the midposition (halfway between full adduction and full abduction with the hand above the head). How many degrees of range of motion is this? What combination of movements are you actually measuring? Write instructions (as they would appear in a goniometry manual) for an OT practitioner who wants to measure humeral motion at the glenohumeral joint. (*Comment: The point of this is to help students realize that they can reason through the process if they understand the movement they are measuring. There is little need to memorize the directions for goniometry.*)
- Palpating muscular activity: To palpate muscle activity is to touch and examine with the hands (to "see" with the hands). Without experience, individuals lack the sensitivity to feel and discriminate between different "feels." Keep the following in mind as you develop skills in this area:
  - Always have the individual who is to be palpated relax.
  - Gently place your hands on the skin that lies over the structure you are trying to palpate.

○ Move your hands in a circular motion, in a sense "looking" for the structure of interest.

Now use the following tips as you work with a partner:

○ For palpation of a muscle or tendon, have your partner move very slightly in a direction you know requires the use of the muscle. Actual movement is not necessary because the thought and intention to move causes a palpable muscle contraction. (*Comment: Movement will make it more difficult to feel the muscle contraction.*)

○ Immediately after the command to move, have your partner relax again. This change—from relaxation to contraction to relaxation—facilitates palpation. In other words, feeling one structure among many others is difficult until activation (contraction of the muscle fibers) defines the structure. Remember that our nervous systems function by differentiating—noticing change. Being aware of a constant stimulus is much more difficult.

○ Now palpate the (1) middle deltoid during attempts to abduct the humerus at the glenohumeral joint, (2) lower pectoralis major during attempts to adduct the humerus at the glenohumeral joint, (3) upper pectoralis major during attempts to flex the humerus at the glenohumeral joint near 90 degrees of shoulder flexion, and (4) anterior deltoid during attempts to flex the humerus at the glenohumeral joint.

• Draw the fibers of the middle deltoid, upper and lower trapezius, and serratus anterior as they abduct the humerus at the shoulder and hold it at 90 degrees of abduction. Draw arrows (vectors), beginning at the insertion and directing the arrow parallel to the fibers toward the origin. Remember, the arrowhead indicates direction. In this case, each force pulls its insertion toward its origin, but the deltoid fibers curve around the acromion. For the deltoid the arrow should start with the fibers from the insertion and continue straight past the point at which the fibers turn. The length of each arrow indicates the strength of contraction. (*Comment: This is difficult for students. They typically need help reviewing attachments so they know where to begin and direct their vectors. It may help to draw the muscle onto the drawing. Then encourage them to simply place the pen on the insertion and begin drawing a straight line through the fibers. You may arbitrarily assign a force amount to each contraction to include the idea of amounts of force being indicated by the length of the vector according to some agreed-upon scale.*)

Exam Questions

1. As a movement at a joint occurs, at what angle of pull is *all* of the force of the muscle being used for rotation?
   a. 45 degrees
   b. 70 degrees
   c. 90 degrees
   d. 120 degrees

2. In terms of angle of pull, where in the motion is the moment arm the longest?
   a. Beginning
   b. End
   c. At an angle of pull of 90 degrees
   d. Exact middle

3. Why can the torque curve not tell us individual flexion tendencies of biceps and brachialis?
   a. It only measures the combined effect of all elbow flexors
   b. Biceps and brachialis never act together in elbow flexion
   c. It measures only those muscles the individual chooses to use
   d. None of the above

4. Scapulohumeral rhythm in raising the hand above the head refers to
   a. Upward scapular rotation combined with glenohumeral (GH) abduction
   b. The combination of proportional amounts of downward scapular rotation and GH abduction
   c. A regular knocking sound occurring with scapular rotation

5. What are the plane and axis for GH abduction?
   a. Sagittal plane; side-to-side axis
   b. Frontal plane; side-to-side axis
   c. Sagittal plane; front-to-back axis
   d. Frontal plane; front-to-back axis

6. Slight downward scapular rotation from paralysis of the upward scapular rotators may cause
   a. Winging of the scapula
   b. Subluxation of the humeral head
   c. Nothing—this is the normal position

7. The subscapularis, infraspinatus, and teres minor are active in
   a. Balancing the upward pull of deltoid on GH joint
   b. Stabilization of the humeral head into the glenoid when holding weight in the hand
   c. Abducting the humerus—last few degrees

8. An individual with weak glenohumeral abductors may abduct the humerus only after externally rotating it. Why?
   a. The individual is using gravity to abduct the humerus
   b. External rotation provides better moment arm for the deltoid
   c. External rotation allows the biceps long head to pull lateral to the abduction axis

9. The elbow joint includes a
   a. Condyloid joint and a hinge joint
   b. Modified ball and socket joint and a hinge joint
   c. Modified hinge joint and a true ball and socket joint

10. Activity in the biceps during elbow extension indicates that the
    a. Biceps is eccentrically contracting
    b. Biceps is concentrically contracting
    c. Biceps is isometrically contracting
    d. None of the above—biceps is never active while the elbow is extending—biceps is a flexor

11. The position for active insufficiency for the biceps is
    a. Elbow flexion and supination
    b. Shoulder extension and abduction and elbow flexion
    c. Shoulder flexion, elbow flexion, and supination
    d. Shoulder flexion and external rotation with supination

12. Pronation and supination require
    a. Rotation of the ulna at the elbow
    b. Abduction of the radius away from the ulna
    c. Rotation of the radius at the elbow
    d. Radial rotation around the ulna proximally

13. In equilibrium of torques during *passive* elbow extension, 10 pounds of pull at the wrist by the OT practitioner equals
    a. Over 100 pounds of active effort by the client
    b. Around 100 pounds of passive tension in the biceps
    c. Something close to 10 pounds of stretch of the biceps in the direction of extension

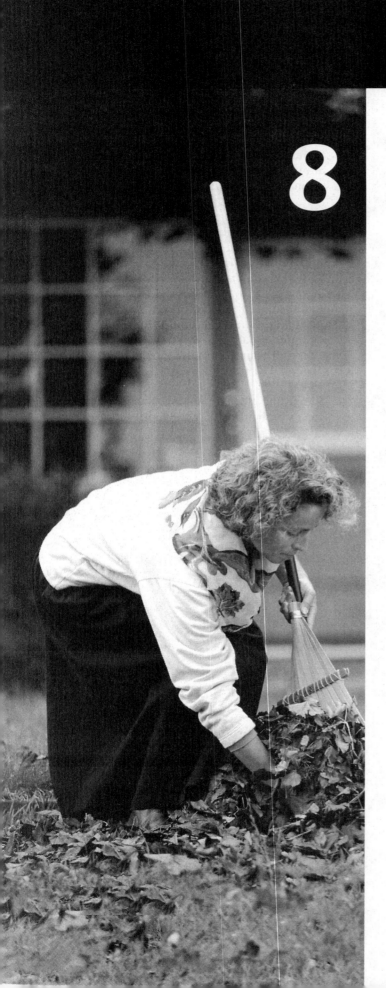

8 The Distal Upper Extremity

CHAPTER **SUMMARY**

he wrist and hand are amazing structures. Watching how they work clarifies and elaborates on our anatomical knowledge. We see that muscle balance at the wrist and metacarpophalangeal (MCP) joints is critical for function. Grasp and manipulation require even more complex systems of balance. Unless many muscles work together, hand function falters. Basic concepts of hand kinesiology make a foundation for clinical diagnosis and treatment.

Learning Objectives

- Describe the differential effects of the major wrist flexors in terms of their functions of wrist flexion with deviation and wrist extension with deviation.
- Identify the strongest function, based on moment arm, of each wrist flexor and extensor.
- Describe how synergistic actions of wrist flexors and extensors yield balanced wrist ulnar and radial deviation.
- Describe the various imbalances at the wrist resulting from radial, ulnar, and median nerve damage at the level of the elbow.
- Explain the basic functions of the extrinsic and intrinsic musculature of the hand.
- Describe the balancing effect of the intrinsics on the long digital extensors.
- List in sequence the intrinsic and extrinsic muscles involved in opening and closing of the hand.
- Describe the effects of ulnar and median nerve damage in opening and closing of the hand.
- Describe the various prehension patterns of the thumb.
- Describe the effect of median and ulnar nerve damage on prehension.
- Identify which grasps require the thumb (and in what capacity) and which do not.
- Describe the differential functions of the thumb carpometacarpal, metacarpophalangeal, and interphalangeal joints.
- Describe the differential uses of the thenar and intrinsic thumb adductor muscles in wide versus narrow grip-span grasps that use the thumb.
- Describe the pathokinesiology of ulnar drift, boutonniere, bowstringing, wrist drop with grip failure, and intrinsic minus hand.
- Differentiate between joint contracture and tendon adhesion, using differential movements of adjacent joints to create slack.
- Explain the basis of tenodesis grip (tendon action) and explain tenodesis using the concept of passive insufficiency.

Laboratory Activities

- Measure MCP hyperextension with traditional goniometry. Normal MCP hyperextension has the feel of a "stiff joint" even though it is normal. Work in a group of at least four people and choose to measure one person using a goniometer:

  - Measure the extent of hyperextension of the index finger's MCP joint. Each of the three measurers must keep their measurements a secret from the other members of the group.
  - Compare the three measurements, which most likely are different. What accounts for these differences? Ask the individual measured whether that individual noticed any difference in the manner in which each measurer performed the measurements. (*Comment: Measurements typically differ based on how much force the measurer uses to range the joint. The point to make is this—controlling that force through torque range of motion techniques [that is, use of a force gauge] allows the measurement to be more objective. This should be demonstrated by the following activity.*)

- For torque range of motion, work with a group of three students to measure MCP hyperextension. While one student uses a goniometer and a force gauge to perform the measurement on a second student, the third student charts the amount of force necessary to hyperextend the MCP to 5 and 10 degrees hyperextension and to the end of its range if that range is beyond 10 degrees. The student should chart measurements on a graph labeled similar to the following:

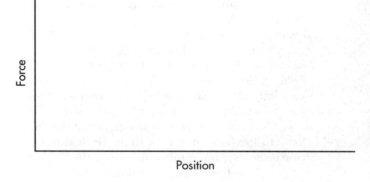

- Look around the classroom and find objects that require the various grasp patterns—cylindrical, spherical, palmar, lateral, hook, power, scissor (thumb adduction), and tip prehension. Use a *T* to indicate which grasps require thumb use and indicate with a *T - O* which require thumb opposition.
- Discuss explanations for the following examples of function after nerve damage. Base your reasoning on a system of thought in which muscles are classified as either "working" or "not working." (*Comment: Have the students read through "working" and "not working" for*

each example of nerve damage. Tell them not to look at the "result" but to justify it before reading this.)

1. Radial nerve damage at elbow, attempted radial deviation:
   Working: Flexor carpi radialis
   Not working: Extensor carpi radialis longus and brevis
   Result: Limited radial deviation with flexion because radial deviation is difficult to perform when the wrist flexes, which occurs when the flexor carpi radialis contracts

2. Radial nerve damage at elbow, attempted wrist flexion:
   Working: Flexor carpi radialis, flexor carpi ulnaris
   Not working: All extensors
   Result: Pure wrist flexion

3. Radial nerve damage above supinator, attempted slow supination without elbow flexion (that is, without intentional elbow flexion):
   Working: Biceps as a supinator
   Not working: Supinator, brachioradialis
   Result: Forearm supination followed by elbow flexion because biceps is being used to supinate

4. Ulnar nerve damage above elbow, attempted ulnar deviation:
   Working: Extensor carpi ulnaris
   Not working: Flexor carpi ulnaris
   Result: Ulnar deviation with extension because the action of the extensor carpi ulnaris (which extends and ulnarly deviates) is unbalanced

5. Median and ulnar nerves damaged at the wrist, attempted full digital extension:
   Working: Extensor digitorum, which extends MCP and interphalangeal (IP) joints of digits
   Not working: All lumbricals, all interossei
   Result: "Clawing" of the digits (MCP hyperextension, slight IP flexion) because action of extensor digitorum is unbalanced without lumbricals or interossei to prevent MCP hyperextension at the end of the full extension sweep; slight IP flexion because interossei and lumbricals extend the IP's (or prevent slight flexion at the end of the sweep)

6. Radial nerve damage above the level of the elbow, attempted digital extension:
   Working: Interossei and lumbricals, wrist flexors (synergists for opening the hand)
   Not working: All extensors of the digits and wrist
   Result: Hand in typical "wrist drop" position; IP extension possible through interossei and lumbricals but accompanied by MCP flexion; simultaneous IP and MCP extension impossible, preventing full hand opening; positioning of the hand to prepare to grasp an object also impossible without wrist ex-

tensors (wrist position normally extended to about 30 or 40 degrees when hand prepares to grasp)

7. Median nerve at the elbow, attempted power grip:
   Working: Interossei and lumbricals to digits 4 and 5, wrist extensors (as synergists), flexor digitorum profundus to digits 4 and 5, and adductor pollicis
   Not working: Flexor digitorum superficialis, flexor digitorum profundus, and lumbricals to digits 2 and 3; abductor pollicis brevis, flexor pollicis brevis, and opponens pollicis (thenars)
   Result: Weak grip using the ulnar side of the hand; digits 2 and 3 attempt to flex around object at MCPs; however, this action is via the interossei, so the IP is extended simultaneously; inability to bring the thumb around (oppose) to firmly lock the object into the palm (if the thumb placed passively, the adductors help hold the object into the palm)

8. Median nerve at the wrist, attempted spherical or cylindrical grasp:
   Working: Flexor digitorum superficialis to all digits, flexor digitorum profundus to all digits, all interossei, lumbricals to digits 4 and 5, flexor pollicis longus and adductor pollicis
   Not working: Lumbricals to digits 2 and 3, all three thenar muscles
   Result: No ability to position thumb in opposition (around the cylinder or ball); thumb in flat position on the plane of the palm; thumb adductor (adductor pollicis) able to adduct thumb against ball or cylinder if thumb is passively placed; slight tendency toward clawing of index and long fingers (digits 2 and 3) but interossei to these two digits preventing full claw; normal appearance in grasp of ulnar side of the hand (digits 4 and 5) but overall grip strength decreased because of failure of radial side of the hand (poorly balanced flexion of digits 2 and 3 and lack of function of thenar muscles)

Exam Questions

1. The wrist joint moves in the sagittal plane for
   a. Abduction/adduction
   b. Flexion/extension
   c. Circumduction

2. The wrist joint is classified as
   a. Ball and socket
   b. Condyloid
   c. Pivot
   d. Saddle

3. Sagittal plane movements of the wrist occur around
   a. One front-to-back axis
   b. Two side-to-side axes
   c. Two front-to-back axes

4. *Balanced* wrist ulnar deviation occurs by way of contractions of
   a. Both the radial and ulnar deviator on the flexor side (anterior) of the wrist side to side axis
   b. The flexor carpi radialis and extensor carpi radialis longus and brevis
   c. The flexor carpi ulnaris and extensor carpi ulnaris

5. Is it possible to purely flex the wrist (without deviation, and without flexing the fingers) with the contraction of only one muscle?
   a. No—each wrist flexor also deviates if contracting alone
   b. Yes—by way of the flexor carpi radialis
   c. Yes—by way of the flexor carpi ulnaris

6. An individual who loses the function of the flexor carpi ulnaris will experience
   a. Weakened wrist extension only
   b. Normal wrist extension but absence of ulnar deviation
   c. Weakened wrist flexion only
   d. Unbalanced/weakened wrist flexion

7. Complete median nerve damage *above the elbow* (affecting innervation to hand intrinsics and extrinsics and wrist muscles) will result in
   a. Weakened wrist flexion that occurs only with radial deviation
   b. Weakened and unbalanced ulnar deviation
   c. Total lack of wrist flexion
   d. Weakened and unbalanced wrist flexion

8. Complete radial nerve damage *at the wrist* will result in which of the following movement (motor) impairments?
   a. None—no motor impairment
   b. Weak wrist flexion
   c. Lack of wrist extension
   d. Impaired grip resulting from lack of wrist extensors

9. Complete radial nerve damage *above the elbow* will result in which of the following movement (motor) impairments?
   a. Lack of wrist flexion
   b. Weak wrist extension—still possible by way of the extensor digitorum communis
   c. Impaired grip
   d. Lack of IP extension

10. Complete ulnar nerve damage *above the elbow* will result in
    a. Ulnar deviation accompanying wrist flexion when trying to flex the wrist
    b. Wrist extension with ulnar deviation when try to ulnarly deviate
    c. Unchanged (normal) ulnar deviation

11. Based on relative lengths of moment arms of the various muscle tendons functioning across the wrist, which of the following is *false*?
    a. Flexor carpi radialis is a better flexor than a radial deviator
    b. Extensor carpi radialis brevis has more deviation effect than extensor carpi radialis longus
    c. Extensor carpi ulnaris has a greater deviator effect than its extensor effect
    d. Flexor carpi ulnaris is better as a flexor than a deviator

12. Considering the five major wrist muscles, which of the following has the *least* tendency toward having a dual function (flexion or extension and deviation)?
    a. Extensor carpi ulnaris
    b. Extensor carpi radialis brevis
    c. Flexor carpi ulnaris
    d. Extensor carpi radialis longus

13. The *best* moment arm for radial deviation occurs with the
    a. ECRL
    b. EPB
    c. FCR
    d. ECU

14. The lumbricals and interossei in *closing the hand* result in
    a. Early flexion of the IPs—shallow digital sweep
    b. Early MCP flexion—providing deep digital sweep
    c. Balancing the pull of the extensor digitorum and preventing MCP hyperflexion
    d. Balancing simultaneous pull of flexor digitorum profundus and extensor digitorum, preventing IP hyperextension

15. Actively flexing the wrist and fingers (all joints simultaneously) results in
    a. Active insufficiency (AI) of the flexors and passive insufficiency (PI) of the extensors
    b. PI of the flexors and AI of the extensors
    c. The best position for creating maximum force in the finger flexors
    d. The most slack position of the extensors

16. Wrist and finger positions corresponding to tenodesis release
    a. Fingers and wrist both flexed
    b. Fingers flexed, wrist slightly extended
    c. Fingers extended, wrist flexed
    d. Fingers and wrist fully extended

17. If an individual *with no functioning nerve supply* to the finger or wrist extensors, releases an object from an "active" grip, you will observe
    a. Active wrist extension and tendon action of the finger flexors
    b. Active or passive wrist flexion and tendon action of the finger extensors
    c. Passive wrist extension and tendon action of the finger extensors
    d. Active wrist flexion and tendon action of the finger flexors

18. An individual *with no functioning nerve supply* to the finger flexors grasps an object. What's happening?
    a. Active wrist flexion and tendon action of the finger extensors
    b. Tension in tendons of the finger flexors after active/passive wrist extension
    c. Wrist extension and active insufficiency of the finger flexors
    d. Wrist flexion and tendon action of the finger flexors

19. A joint contracture on the extensor side of the MCP limits
    a. PIP flexion
    b. MCP flexion
    c. PIP extension
    d. PIP flexion and extension
    e. MCP extension and flexion

20. In the case of surgical shortening of the FDP tendons (tenodesis), MCP and IP flexion contractures can be prevented without stretching the FDP by
    a. Simultaneous wrist and finger extension
    b. Simultaneous MCP and IP extension
    c. Extension of one joint while others are flexed
    d. Extension of all joints but one combined with a maximum contraction of the muscle

21. A grasp *not* requiring opposition of the thumb is the
    a. 3-jaw chuck
    b. Cyndrical grasp
    c. Tip-to-tip prehension between thumb and little finger
    d. Lateral pinch ("key pinch")

22. Which type of thumb use in grasp is still possible after median nerve damage *at the elbow?*
    a. Lateral pinch (*HINT: Where is FPL innervated?*)
    b. Power grasp
    c. Opposition
    d. Scissor—adduction of thumb to the palm

23. In ulnar nerve damage *at the wrist* there is hyperextension of MCPs of digits
    a. 2 and 3—loss of interossei; 4 and 5—loss of 3rd and 4th lumbricals and interossei
    b. 2 and 3—loss of 1st and 2nd lumbricals
    c. 4 and 5—loss of flexor digitorum profundus
    d. 2 to 5—loss of thenars and adductor pollicis

24. Normal thumb grasp *around* a coffee cup requires
    a. Abducted thumb—active adductor pollicis
    b. Thumb opposition—active opponens pollicis only
    c. Abducted thumb—active abductor pollicis brevis
    d. Adducted thumb—active adductor pollicis

25. With radial nerve damage, the fingers exhibit partial extension to open to receive the cup via
    a. Tenodesis grasp
    b. Lumbricals/interossei
    c. Extensor digitorum communis

26. Late in opening the hand the lumbricals and interossei are
    a. Inactive
    b. Active—preventing MCP hyperextension
    c. Active—providing slight IP flexion at the end of the extension sweep
    d. Active—providing shallow digital sweep into extension

27. In boutonniere, the torn extensor aponeurosis (extensor hood) slips
    a. Dorsally—behind the PIP F/E axis
    b. Volarly—in front of the PIP F/E axis
    c. Laterally—to the ulnar side of the MCP abduction/adduction axis
    d. Laterally—the ulnar side of the PIP abduction/adduction axis

28. Again, in boutonniere, the new position results in inability to actively
    a. Extend the MCP
    b. Flex the PIP
    c. Extend the PIP
    d. Extend any joints in the finger

29. In ulnar "drift" of the MCP ("wind swept hand"),
    a. Tendons of the FDP develop a moment arm for deviation of the PIPs
    b. Tendons of the FDS decrease in their moment for MCP flexion
    c. The EDC becomes a flexor of the MCP joints
    d. **Tendons of the EDC develop a moment arm for deviation of the MCP**

30. Palmar abduction of the thumb occurs at which joint(s) and in which plane?
    a. **CMC joint; perpendicular to the plane of the palm**
    b. MCP joint; perpendicular to the plane of the palm
    c. CMC joint; parallel to or on the surface of the palm
    d. MCP and IP joints; parallel to or on the surface of the palm

31. Full flexion and extension of the thumb involves movement at the
    a. **CMC, MCP, and IP joints**
    b. MCP and IP joints only
    c. MCP joint only
    d. CMC joint only

32. Opposition of the thumb has occurred when
    a. The thumb is flexed into the palm opposite the little finger
    b. **There has been rotation of the first metacarpal along with abduction and partial flexion**
    c. The thumb touches any of the other four digits—on any side of the digit
    d. The pad of the thumb touches the radial side of the other digits

33. What motion of the thumb is necessary in cylindrical, spherical, palmar (3-jaw chuck), and fine tip prehension and requires the CMC joint of the thumb?
    a. Flexion
    b. **Opposition**
    c. Extension
    d. Adduction

34. The problem *described by the client* who experiences the typical effect of bowstringing is
    a. **Lack of full motion at the joint**
    b. Intense pain with movement
    c. Extra movement at the joint

35. "Wrist drop" is associated with
    a. Complete inability to extend *any* joint of the fingers
    b. Inability to fully extend the wrist but *ability* to hold the wrist in neutral during function
    c. Passive insufficiency of the finger flexors
    d. **Inability to exert a powerful grasp on an object**

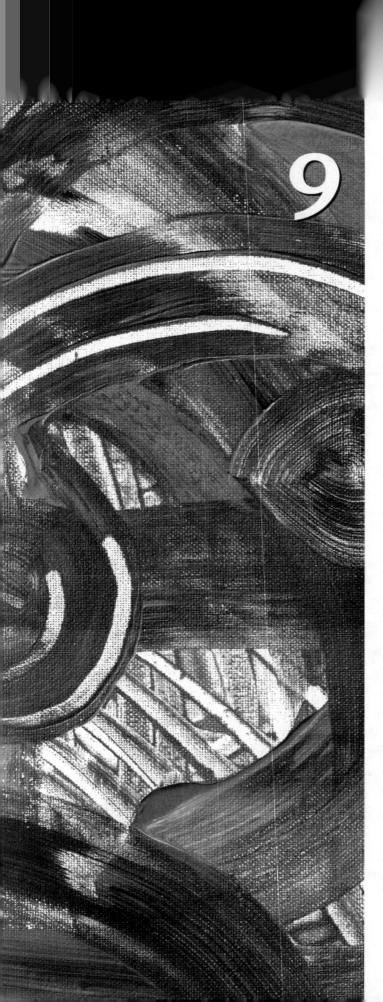

The Lower Extremity

9

CHAPTER **SUMMARY**

Most people associate the lower extremities solely with walking. In many cases walking is an important association, especially after injuries and accidents that impair mobility. Our lower extremities do more than just transport us from place to place. Muscles at the hip produce closed-chain actions that move and position the trunk for reaching tasks. They also balance the trunk at the hip in sitting and maintain the center of gravity projection through the base of support in standing. The weight shifts required in sitting, standing, and walking involve trunk lateral flexion, extension, and forward flexion as well as inclination of the trunk through closed-chain abduction, adduction, flexion, and extension of the hip.

The lower extremities provide us with a base of support for sitting and standing and move us from one base to the next in transfers. When lower extremity function is impaired, wheelchairs serve as a locomotor extension of the trunk. All the same principles of stability apply and are altered largely by the presence and position of lower extremities

Biomechanical analysis provides a tool for understanding function through systematic determination of movements, positions, and muscle activation. Biomechanical analysis concentrates on details, components of movement and positioning, examining the "trees" *after gazing* at the forest. Ultimately, biomechanical analysis and our heightened understanding of the musculoskeletal system through kinesiology serve to enrich our clinical perspective. They allow us better appreciation of the forest. An informed view leads to more effective problem solving. Through adaptation we can transform or reincorporate impaired function so that the tasks essential to role performance keep individuals actively engaged at home and in their community.

Learning Objectives

- List and describe the four factors in stability and identify the missing stability factor in an unstable situation.
- Describe the stability problem of an individual with recent bilateral lower-extremity amputations as the individual attempts to move a wheelchair.
- Identify the stability risks associated with recliner wheelchairs.
- Demonstrate a safe wheelchair-to-bed standing pivot transfer, identifying the original and the new bases of support.
- Describe the lower-extremity movements in the sagittal and frontal planes during normal gait.
- Describe the muscle activity responsible for the movements in the sagittal and frontal planes during normal gait.
- Describe two compensations that an individual with weak hip abductors can use during unilateral stance.

Laboratory Activities

*(**Comment:** Please perform the following activities only if close supervision is available. You may want the students to wear bi-*

cycle helmets for the activities involving wheelchair stability. The publisher and author do not endorse these activities unless they are performed under close supervision and exactly as described.)

- Students should pair up and take turns with this activity. After securing a watchful partner, sit in a wheelchair, remove the legrests, footrests, and arm rests (if removable); and instruct your partner to stand behind you with hands on the handles (canes). Try the following exercises:
  - With your feet hanging toward the ground, use your hands to push the rear wheels forward strongly enough that the front casters rise slightly off the ground. Make sure that your partner's hands remain on the handles and your partner is ready to catch you.
  - If you are unable to lift the front of the chair, instruct your partner to tilt you back slowly so that the front casters are in the air and try to balance the chair yourself. If you sense you are leaning too far backward, pull backward on the wheels (handrails) as if to back up. If you sense you are falling forward (front casters moving toward the ground again), push the rear wheels (handrails) forward to put your chair "back in flight."
  - After 5 minutes, switch roles.
  - Identify the projection of the center of gravity of the seated individual when all four wheels are on the ground and when only the rear (large) wheels are on the ground.
  - In terms of factors of stability, why is a wheelie so hard to achieve and maintain?
- Transfers: Students should pair up and use a wheelchair and a transfer belt to attempt both a sliding board transfer and a stand-pivot transfer. Describe each transfer in terms of base of support and center of gravity projection. *(**Comment:** Please refer to the text for descriptions of the three bases of support involved in transferring and the importance of projection of the center of gravity into the base of support.)*
- Again, get in a wheelchair with your partner spotting you by holding onto the push handles:
  - Attempt a fast start by pushing hard on the rear-wheel rails.
  - Repeat this action but remove the footrests and fold your legs crossed in the seat so that they no longer hang down. Attempt a fast start (after ensuring that your partner is in place). What happens this second time with your legs folded?
- Wheel around in the chair and pull up to a spot. Stop without backing up first and lock the chair:
  - With your feet in the footrests and your partner in

front of you, lean forward, bringing your chest to your knees as if to reach for something on the floor in front of you. What happens as you lean forward?

○ Wheel around again. This time stop and back up about 4 feet and put on the brakes. Lean forward as you did before, with your partner in place. What happens as you lean forward this time?

○ What accounts for the difference in the chair's stability as you lean forward? (*HINT: Think about the front-to-back dimension of the base of support in each case.*)

○ Based on this experience, what is the general rule for coming to a stop if you intend to lean forward?

Exam Questions

1. Balancing the upper body at the hip against the pull of gravity in bilateral standing,
   a. The hip flexors activate if the center of gravity falls anterior to the side-to-side axis
   b. The hip extensors activate if the center of gravity falls anterior to the side-to-side axis

2. You are standing with your humerus fully abducted, hand above your head, raising your cap in celebration! To *slowly lower* the cap back down to your head, you contract
   a. Glenohumeral adductors concentrically
   b. Elbow flexors concentrically
   c. Elbow extensors eccentrically
   d. Glenohumeral abductors concentrically

3. You have learned that your gastroc and soleus muscles (calf muscles) are the agonists for ankle plantar flexion. Stand up and move from flat foot to standing on your toes. This is
   a. Plantar flexion—open-chain
   b. Dorsiflexion—closed-chain
   c. Dorsiflexion—open-chain
   d. Plantar flexion—closed-chain

4. In the previous question the active muscle group and contraction type is
   a. Dorsiflexors—eccentric
   b. Dorsiflexors—concentric
   c. Plantar flexors—concentric
   d. Plantar flexors—eccentric

5. In the gait cycle, what occurs just before toe-off?
   a. Heel strike
   b. Foot flat
   c. Heel off
   d. Toe-fu

6. In the gait cycle, swing occurs immediately before
   a. Toe off
   b. Heel strike
   c. Heel off
   d. Rock-n-roll by about 15 to 20 years (true, but has nothing to do with the gait cycle)

7. In the gait cycle, hip flexion occurs from
   a. Heel strike to heel off (stance, in gait cycle)
   b. Toe off to heel strike (swing, in gait cycle)
   c. Heel strike to heel strike (stance and swing)

8. When hip flexion occurs in the gait cycle, there is concentric contraction of the
   a. Hip flexors
   b. Hip extensors

9. During stance in the gait cycle, an eccentric contraction of the _____ on the weight bearing side allows slight _____.
   a. Hip abductors; open-chain abduction
   b. Hip abductors; closed-chain adduction
   c. Hip adductors; closed-chain abduction
   d. Hip adductors; open-chain adduction

10. In late swing in the gait cycle, knee extension is slowed down by the knee flexors (hamstrings) contracting
    a. Eccentrically
    b. Isometrically
    c. Concentrically

11. A woman leaning forward is _____ stable than the same woman standing straight.
    a. More
    b. Less

12. A woman in high heels is _____ stable than the same woman standing in swim fins.
    a. More
    b. Less

13. A man walking on all fours is _____ stable than the same man walking on two feet.
    a. More
    b. Less

14. A man standing on one foot is _____ stable than a man on two feet because the man on one foot _____.
    a. Less; has a lower center of gravity
    b. Less; has a narrower base of support
    c. More; spends less money on shoes

15. A recliner wheelchair positioned with the back fully reclined may be unstable since the
    a. Projection of the center of gravity is close to the rear edge of the base of support and may be behind it
    b. Center of gravity of the individual in the chair is higher when reclined
    c. Projection of the base of support is close to the rear edge of the center of gravity
    d. Chair now has a lower center of gravity

16. A wheelchair "wheelie" is difficult to maintain because
    a. The size of the base of support continually changes
    b. The center of gravity is too high to be stable
    c. The projection of the center of gravity has such a small base of support within which to fall

17. The hip joint is an example of a _____ and allows motion in _____.
    a. Hinge joint; 3 planes
    b. Ball and socket joint; 2 planes
    c. Pivot joint; 1 plane
    d. Ball and socket joint; 3 planes
    e. Saddle joint; 3 planes

Transparency Masters

The following transparency masters (TMs) were selected from figures in the text thought to be most helpful in the clarification of major points. After lectures, many students ask where they might obtain illustrations used during class. Seeing, in this case, that the instructor used illustrations from the text may help reinforce the usefulness of reading and studying the text required (or recommended) for their course.

Transparency masters list the TM number, the corresponding figure number in the text, and a title. These pages have been perforated for easy removal.

Transparency List

A, Ulnar drift; **B,** Boutonniere; **C,** Swan neck (Figure 2-5)

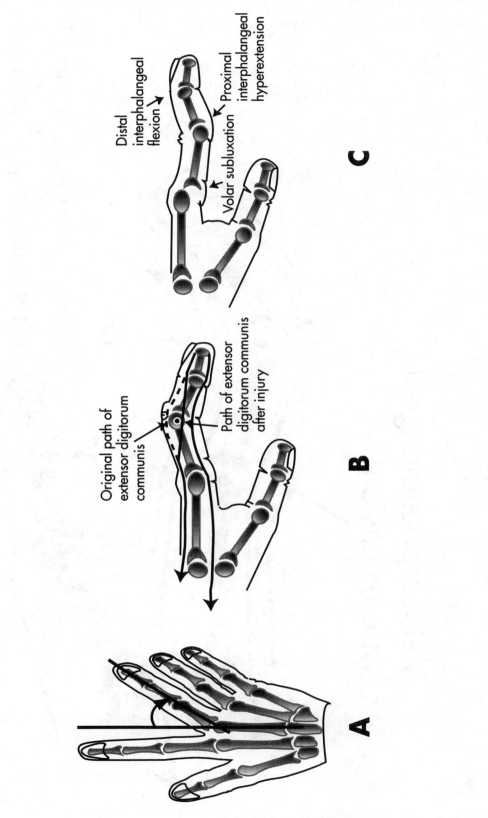

Distal interphalangeal flexion

Proximal interphalangeal hyperextension

Volar subluxation

Original path of extensor digitorum communis

Path of extensor digitorum communis after injury

C

B

A

Greene/Roberts: Kinesiology: Movement in the Context of Activity
Copyright © 1999, Mosby, Inc.

TM 2
Intrinsic minus (Figure 2-6)

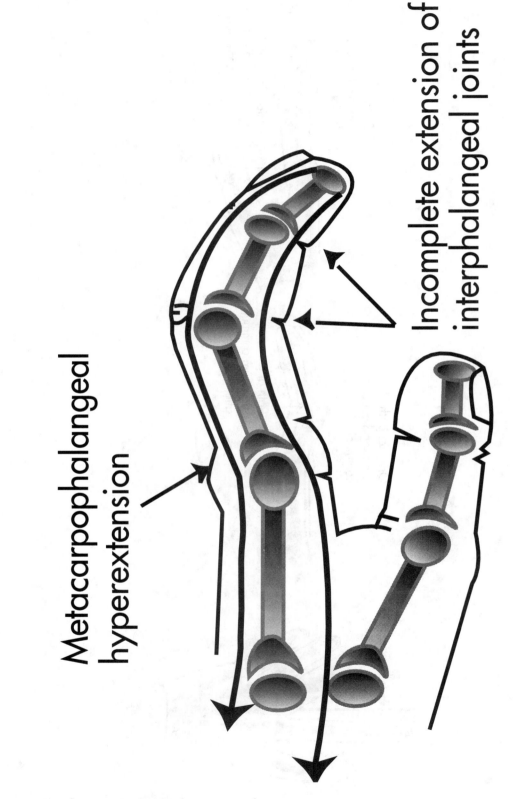

Incomplete extension of interphalangeal joints

Metacarpophalangeal hyperextension

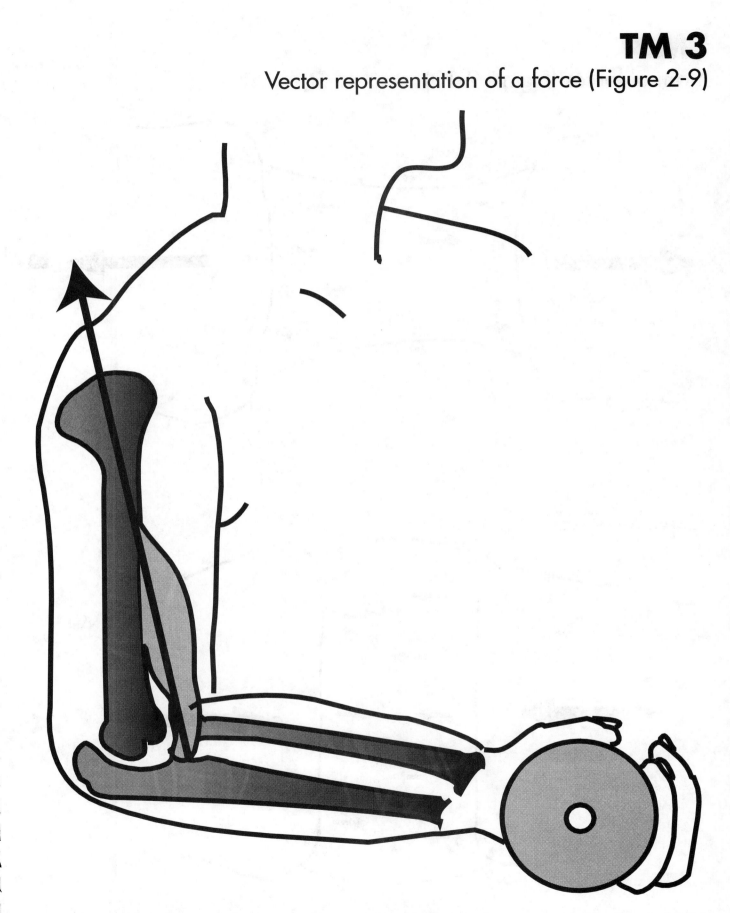

TM 4
Normal forces (Figure 2-10)

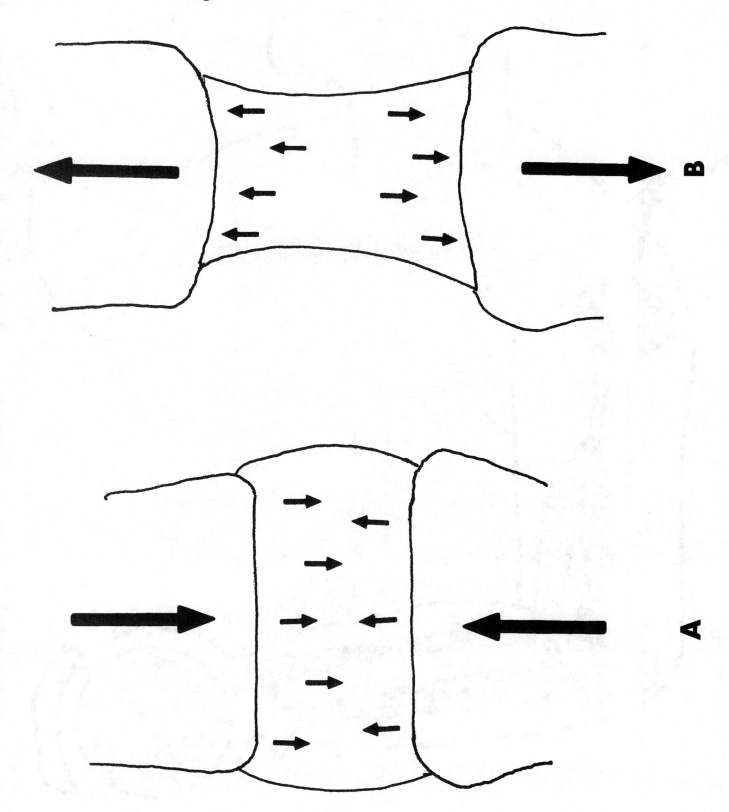

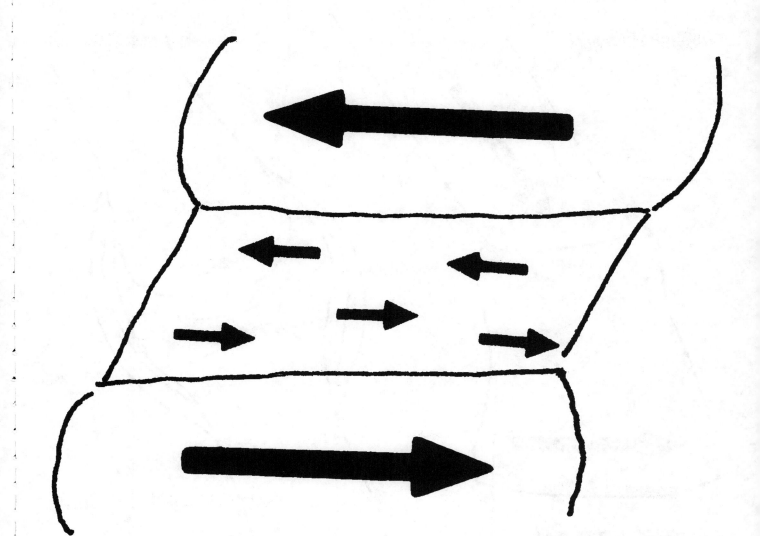

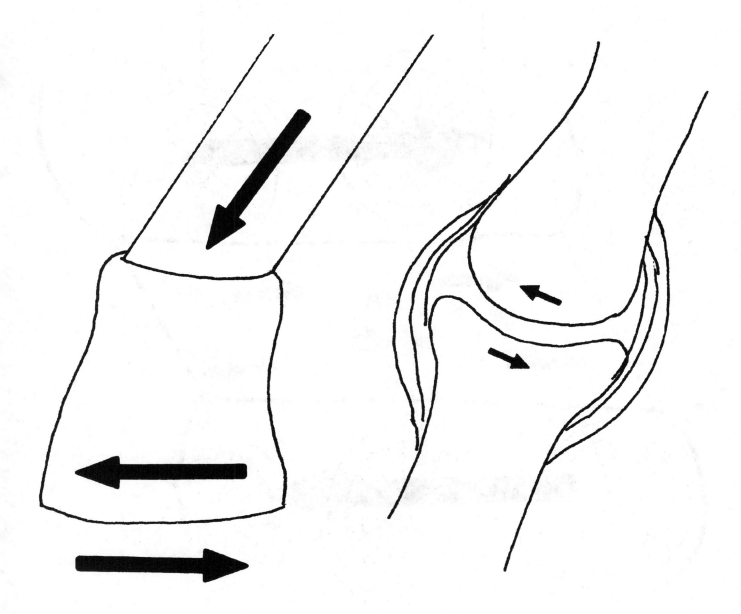

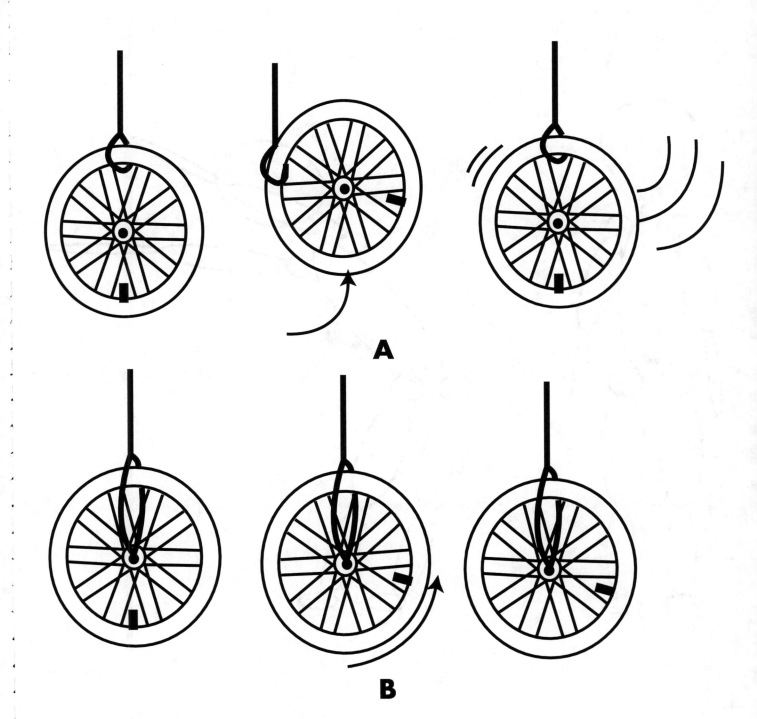

A

B

TM 8

Body position and the center of gravity (Figure 3-3)

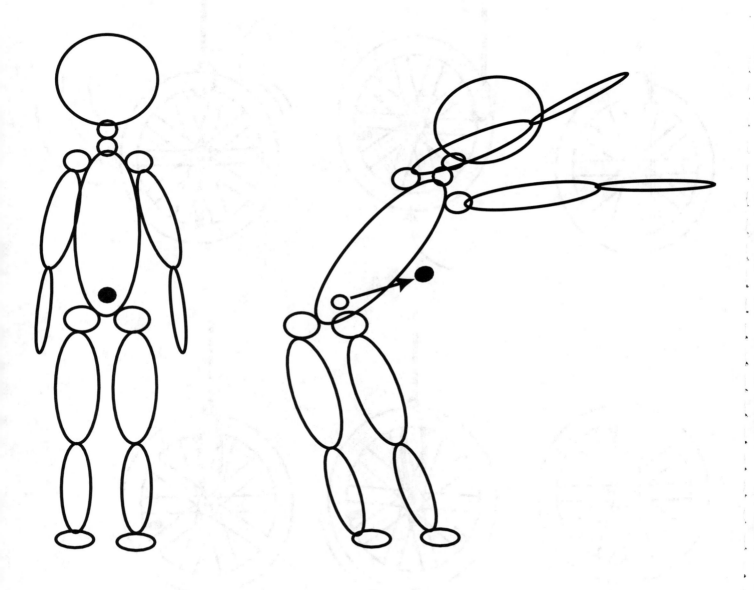

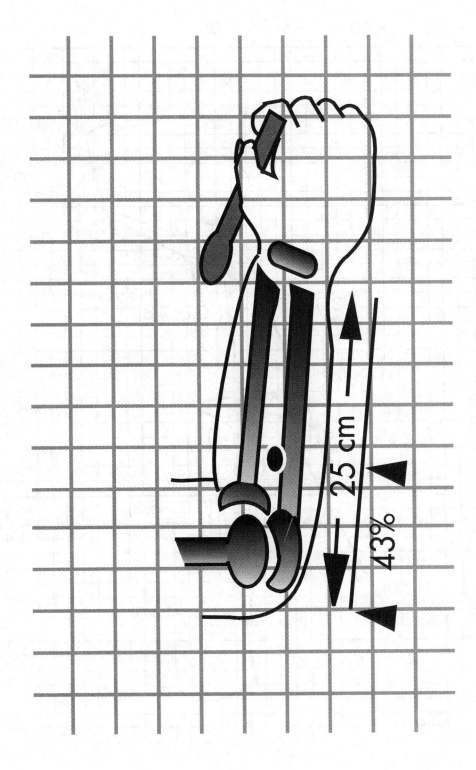

TM 10

Segmental centers of gravity contributing to the center of gravity of the entire person (Figure 3-5, B)

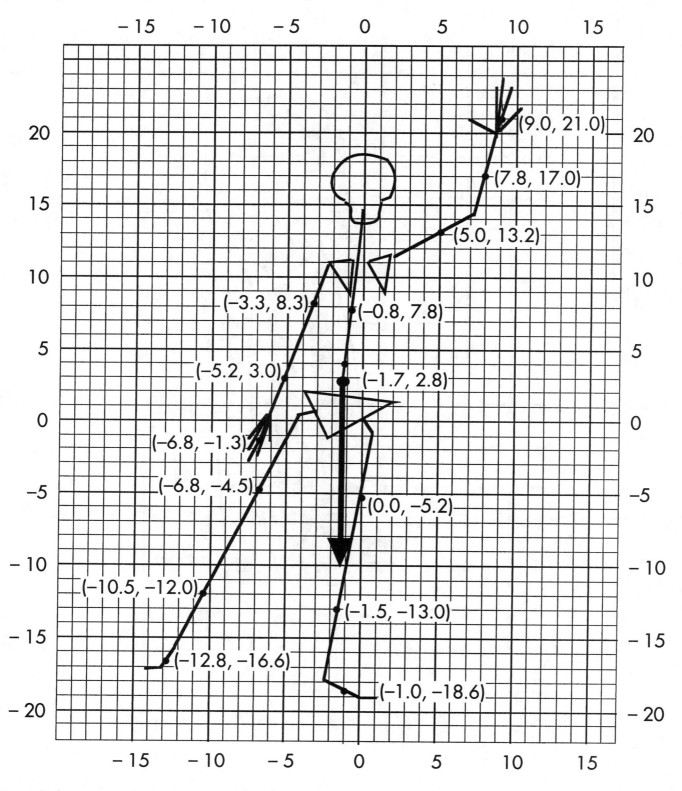

Center of gravity of person seated in a wheelchair (Figure 3-6)

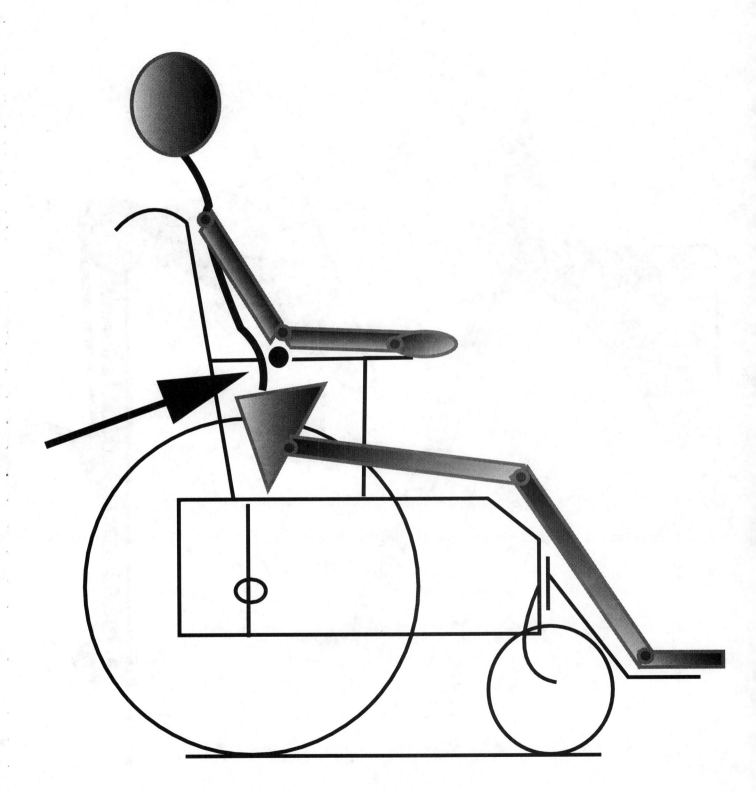

TM 12

Deltoid acting on its insertion (**A**) and origin (**B**) (Figure 4-1)

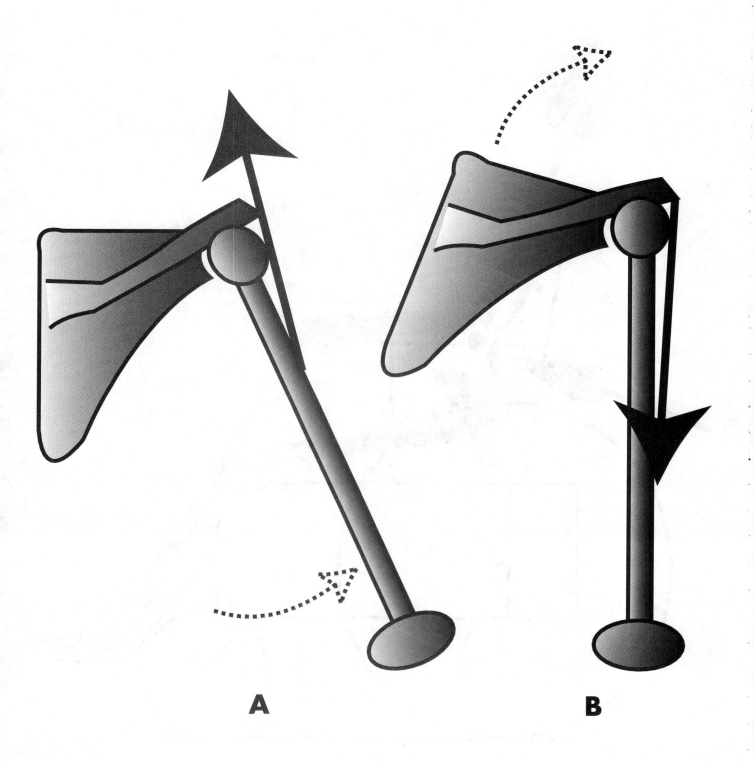

A   **B**

A food server's tray: force equilibrium (Figure 4-2)

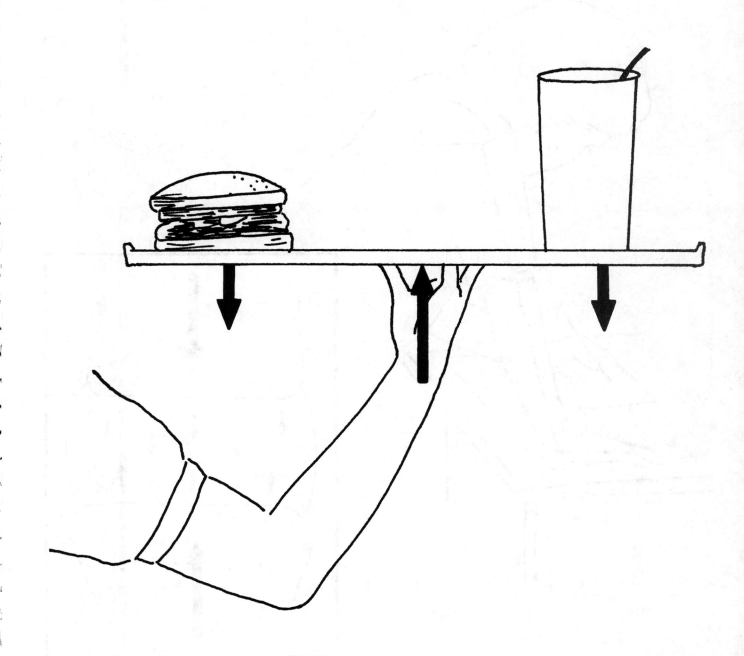

TM 14

Compressive force in leaning on a table (Figure 4-3)

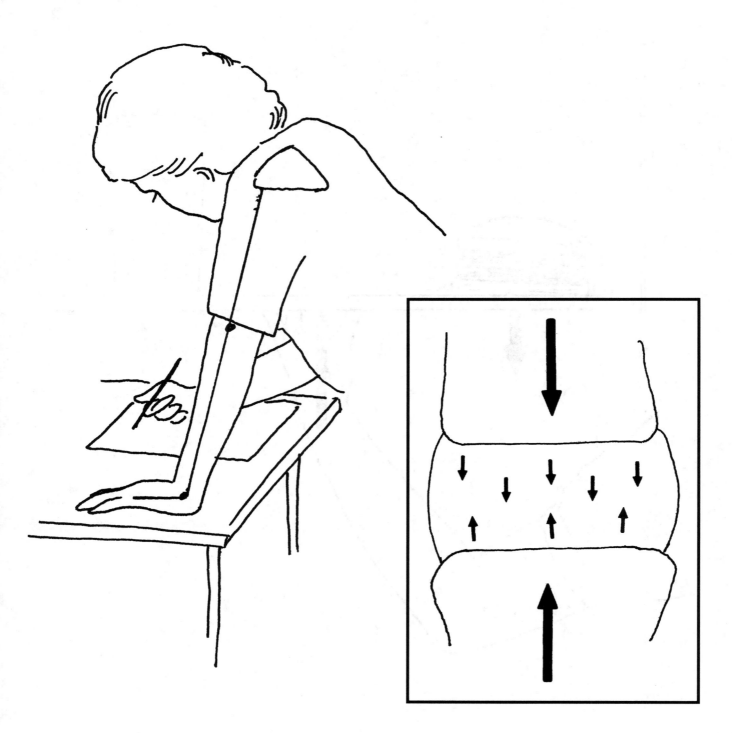

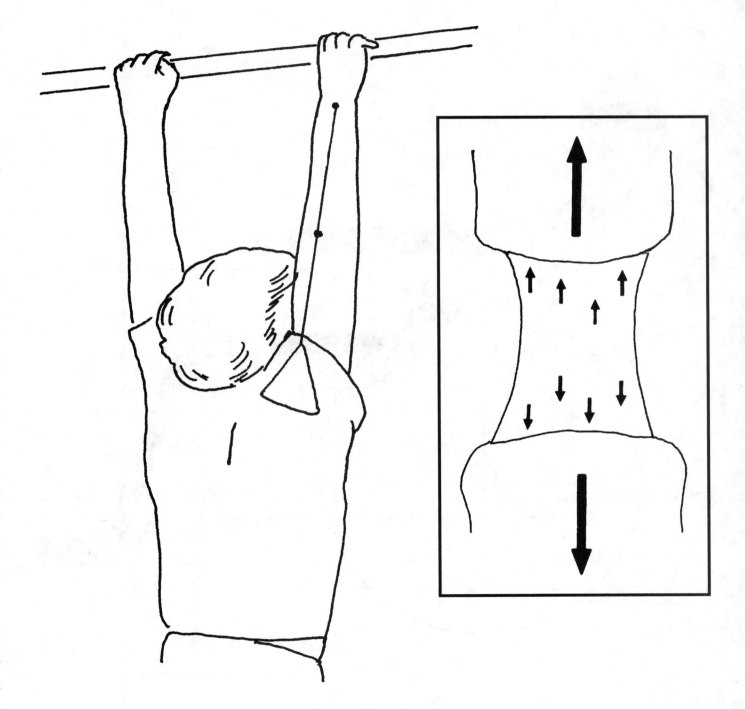

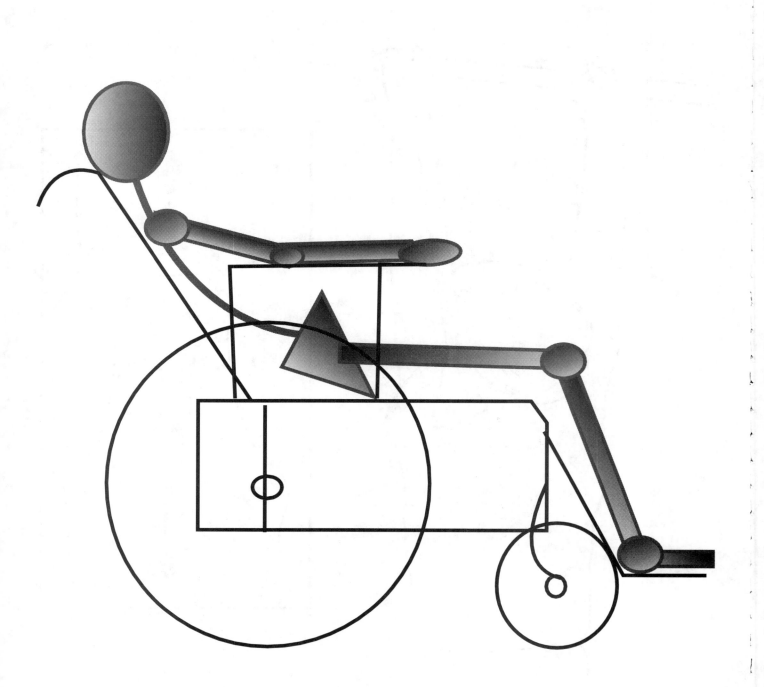

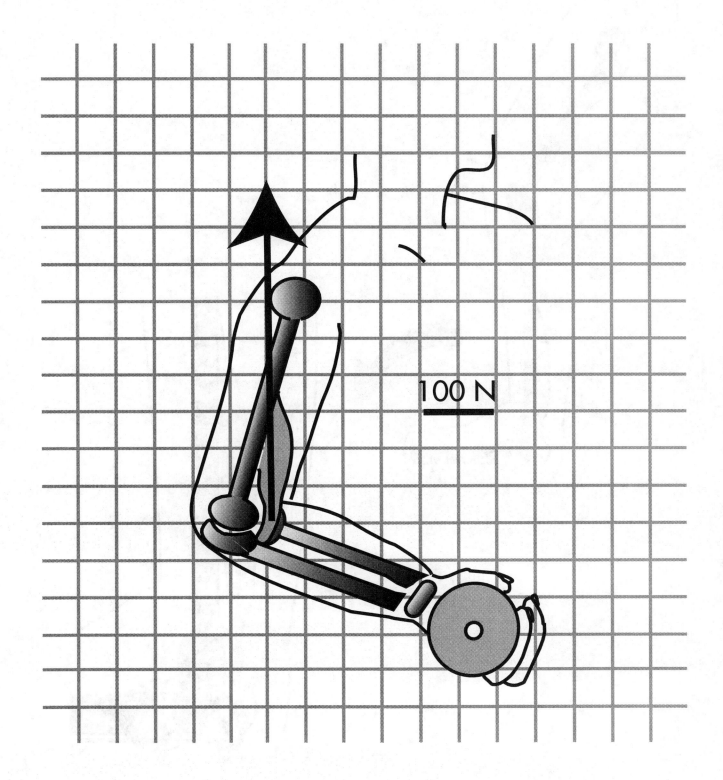

100 N

TM 18
Indicating force direction (Figure 4-7)

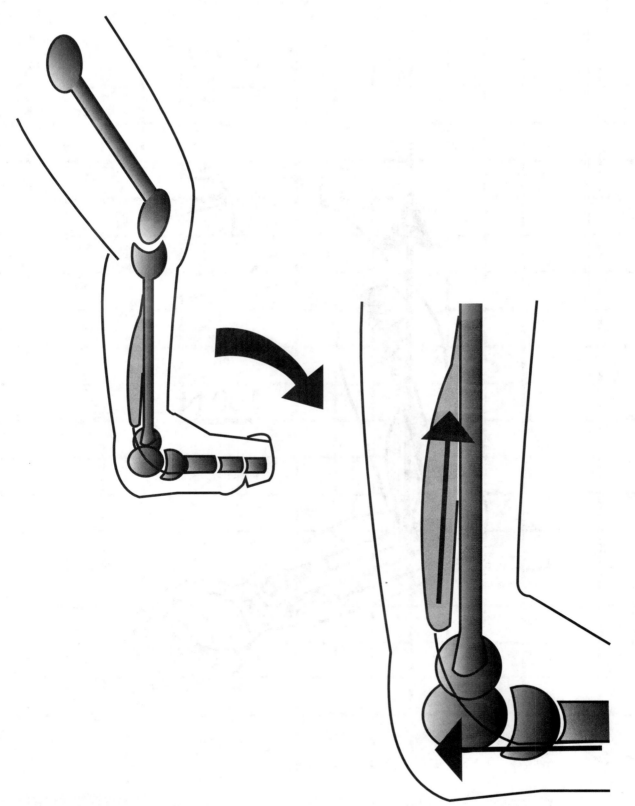

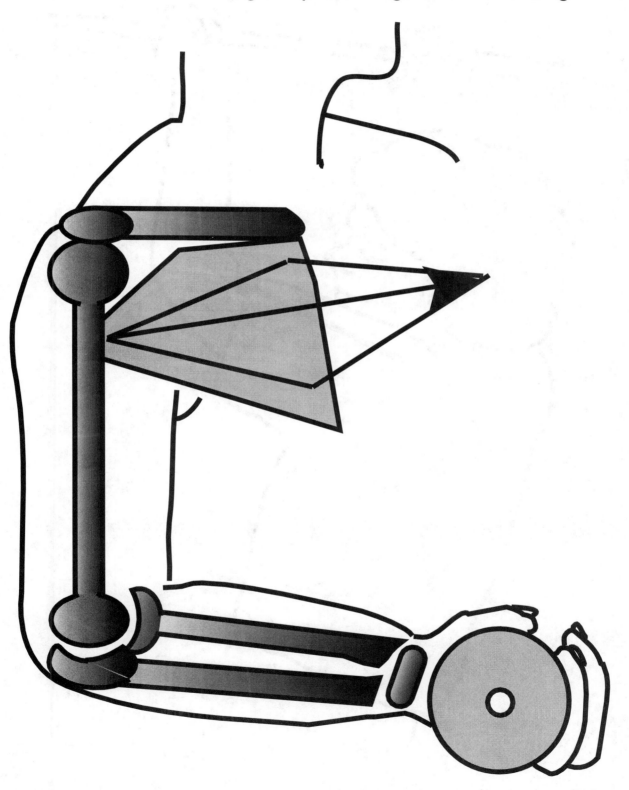

TM 20

Closed-chain elbow flexion (Figure 4-10)

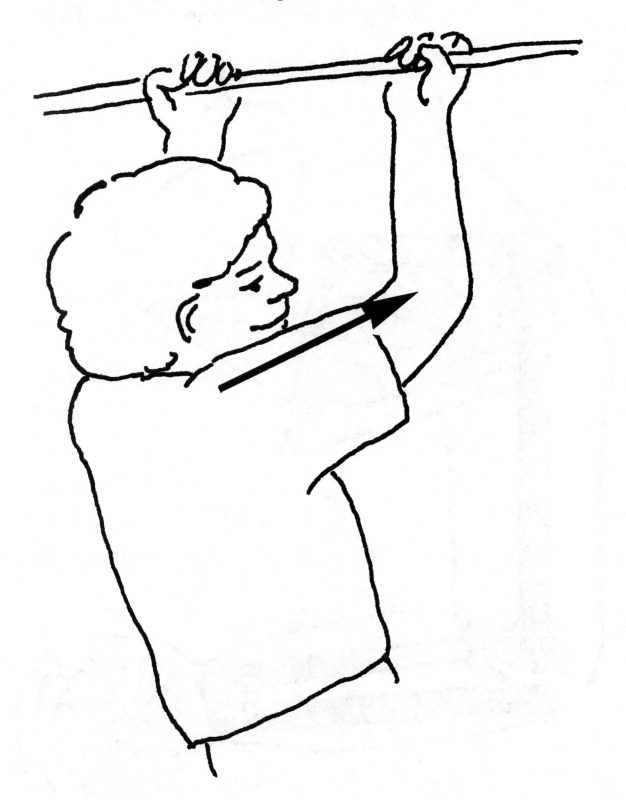

Comparison of fusiform (**A**), and pennate (**B**) muscles (Figure 4-11)

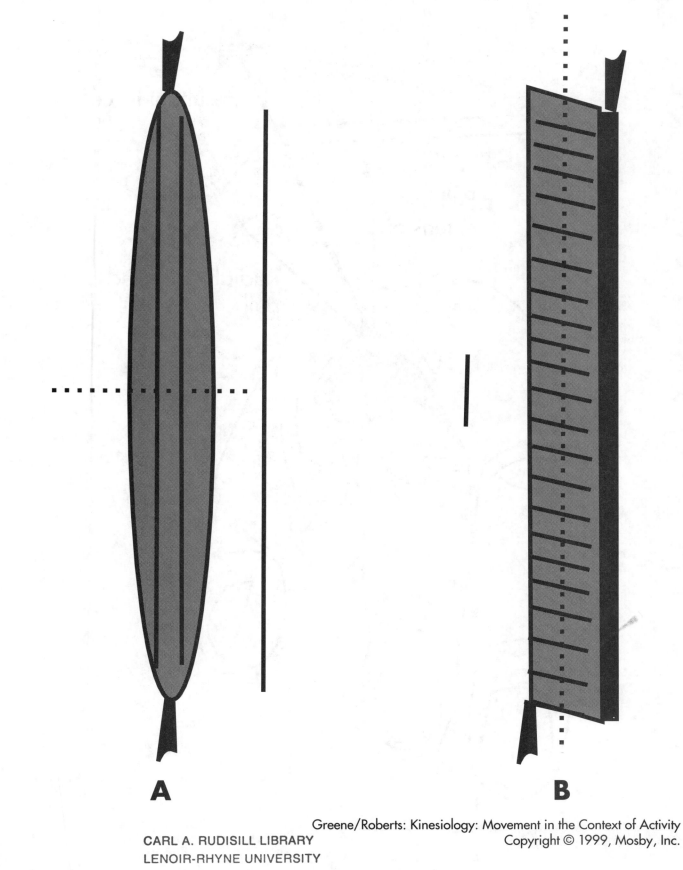

A

B

Greene/Roberts: Kinesiology: Movement in the Context of Activity
Copyright © 1999, Mosby, Inc.

TM 22

Combining forces in splinting to find the resultant (Figure 4-19)

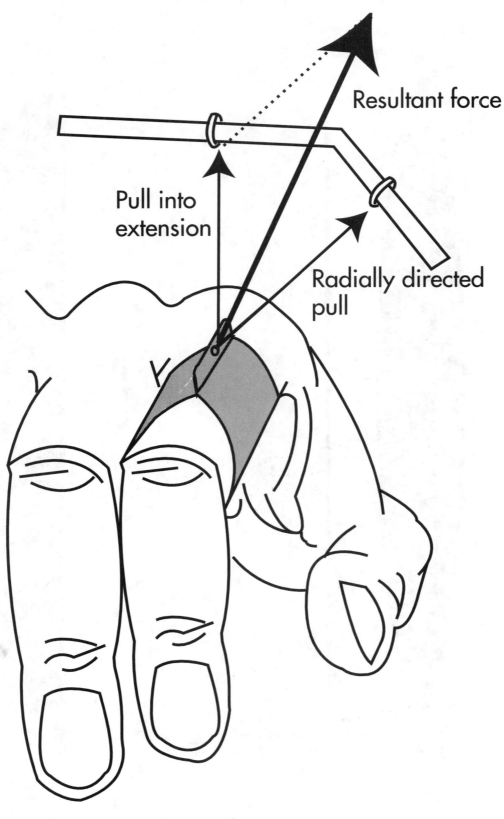

Resultant force

Pull into extension

Radially directed pull

Vector representation of muscle contraction types (Figure C-6)

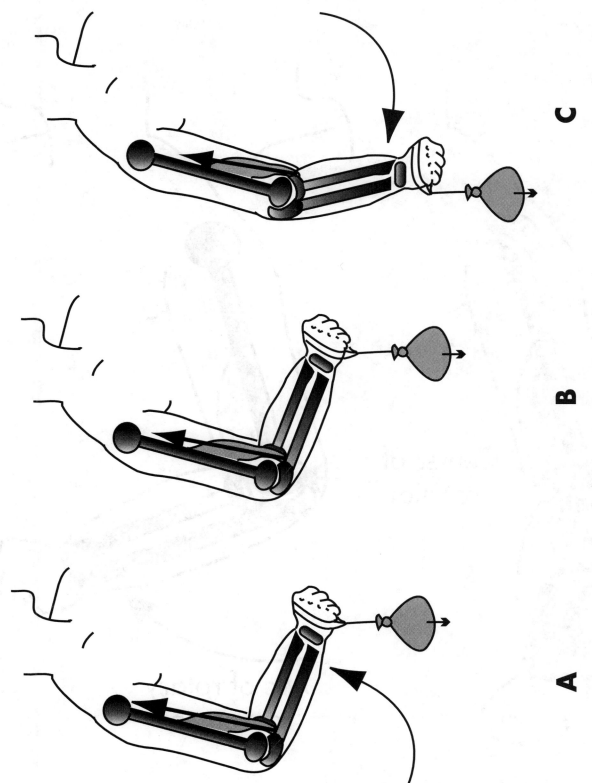

TM 24

Center of rotation for forearm flexion (Figure 5-1)

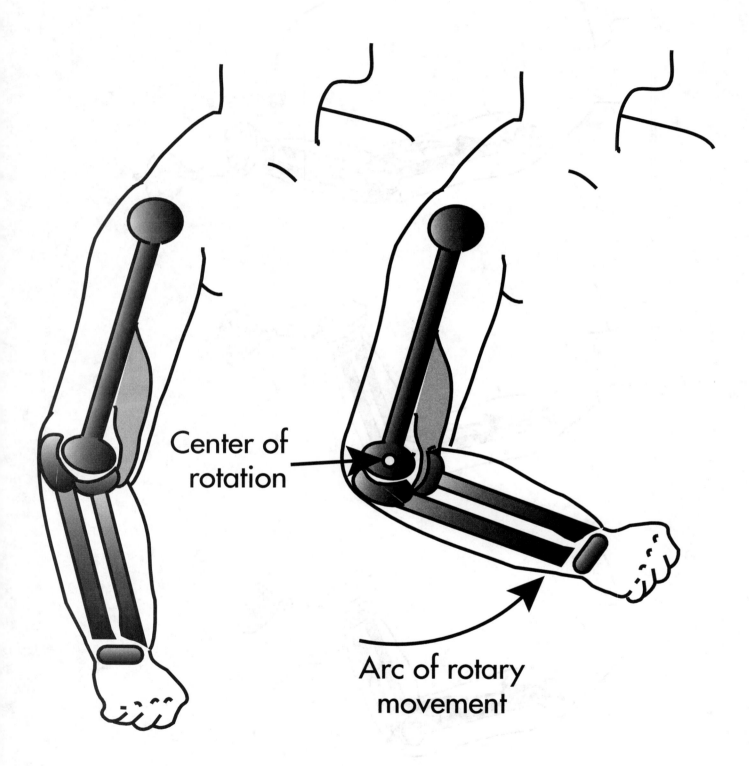

Center of rotation

Arc of rotary movement

TM 25

Fundamental characteristics of rotary motion (Figure 5-2)

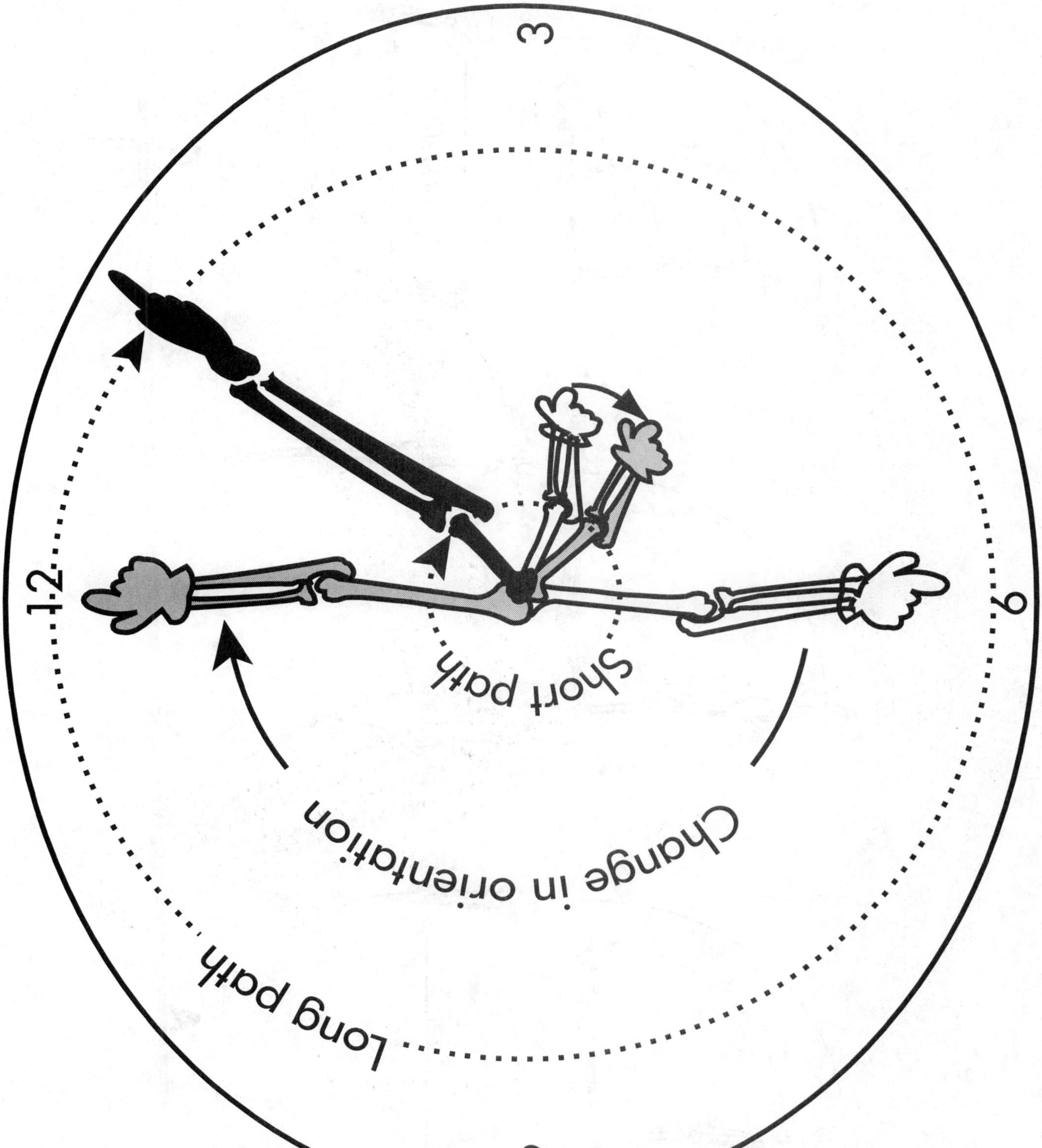

Greene/Roberts: Kinesiology: Movement in the Context of Activity

TM 26

Rotary compared to linear motion (Figure 5-3)

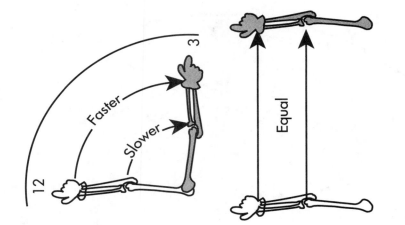

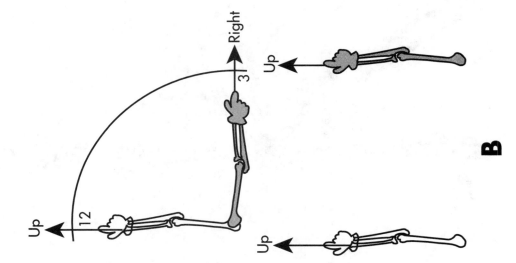

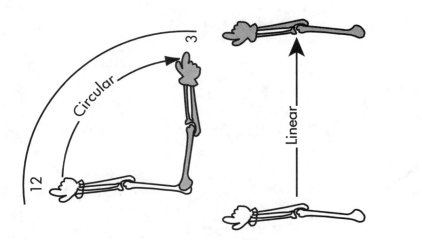

C

B

A

Tendencies toward elbow flexion and extension (Figure 5-4)

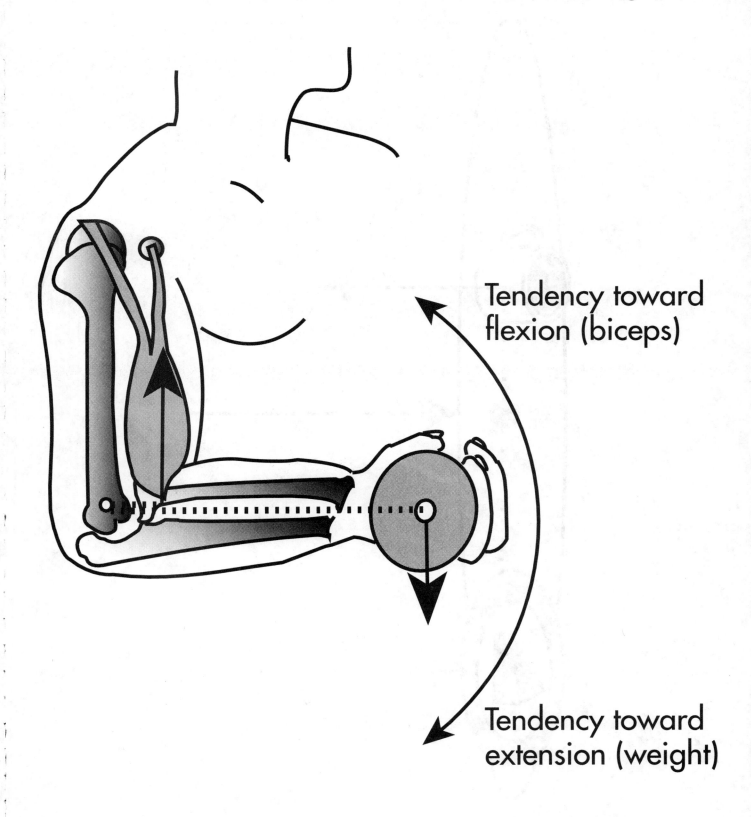

Tendency toward flexion (biceps)

Tendency toward extension (weight)

TM 28

Rotary equilibrium of a food server's tray (Figure 5-5)

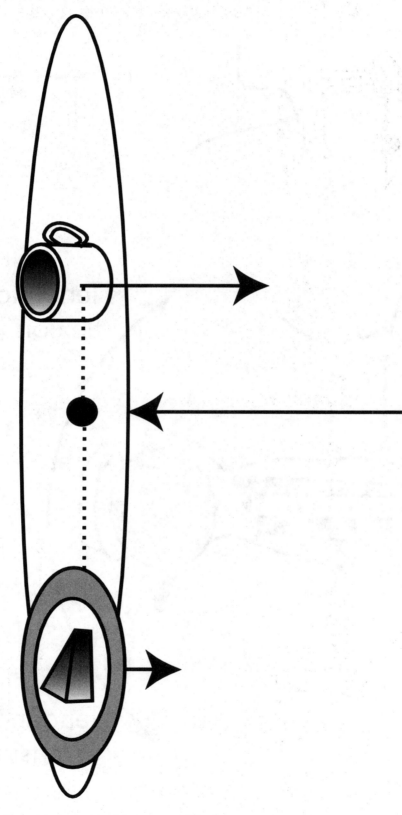

Three classes of levers: **A,** First class; **B,** Second class; **C,** Third class (Unnumbered figures in Table 5-1)

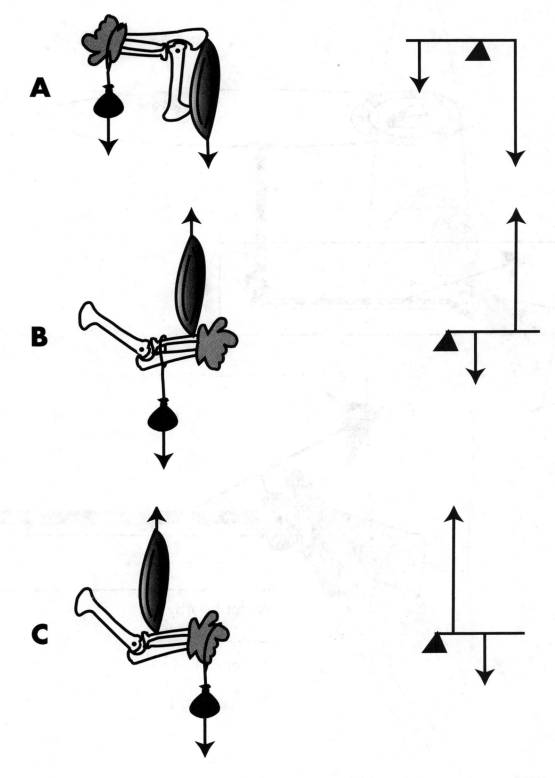

TM 30

Equilibrium of abduction and adduction
torques at the shoulder (Figure 5-10)

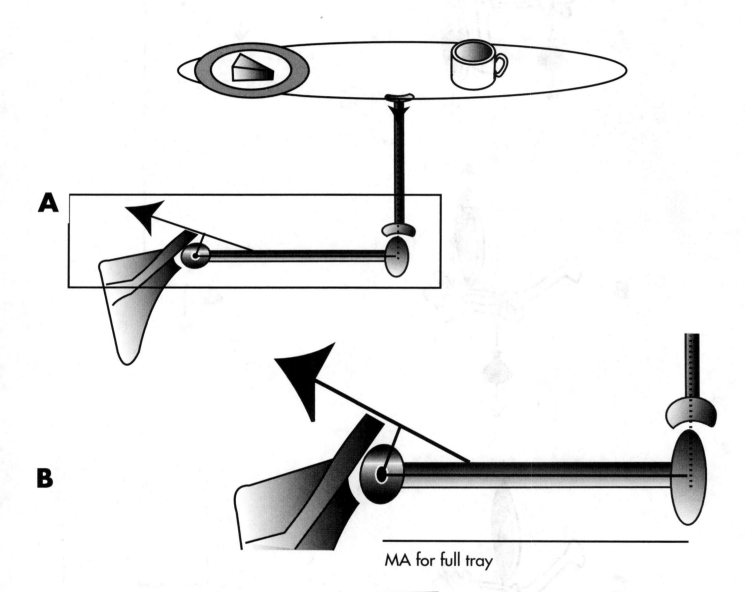

A

B

MA for full tray

MA for deltoid force

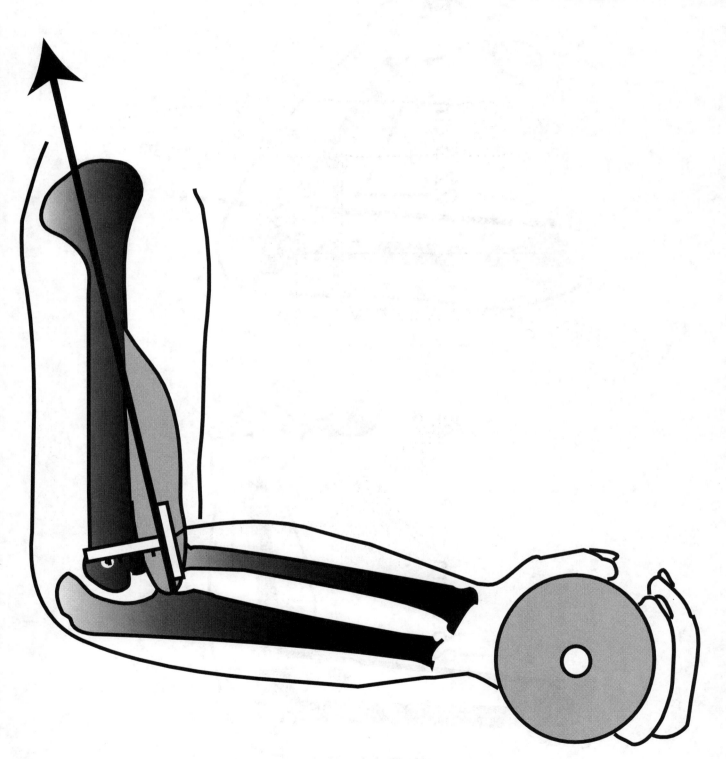

TM 32

Internal torque affected by joint position (Figure 5-14)

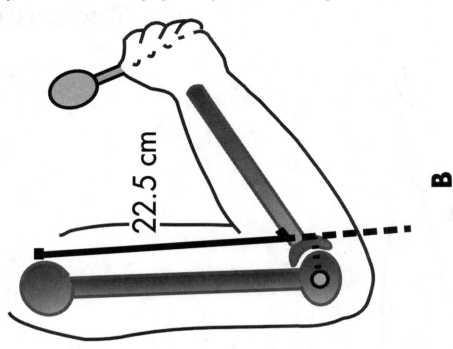

22.5 cm

B

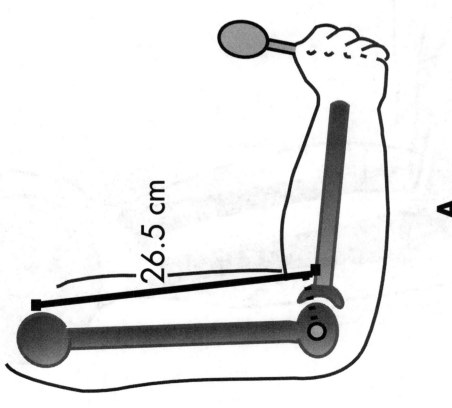

26.5 cm

A

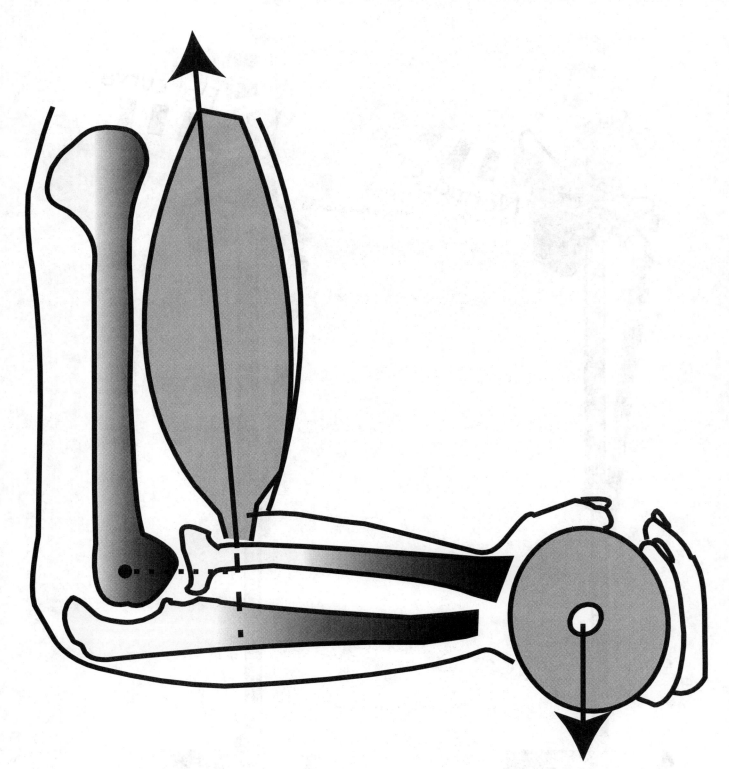

TM 34

Normal vs. short hamstrings, forward bending,
and the vertebral column (Figure 6-3)

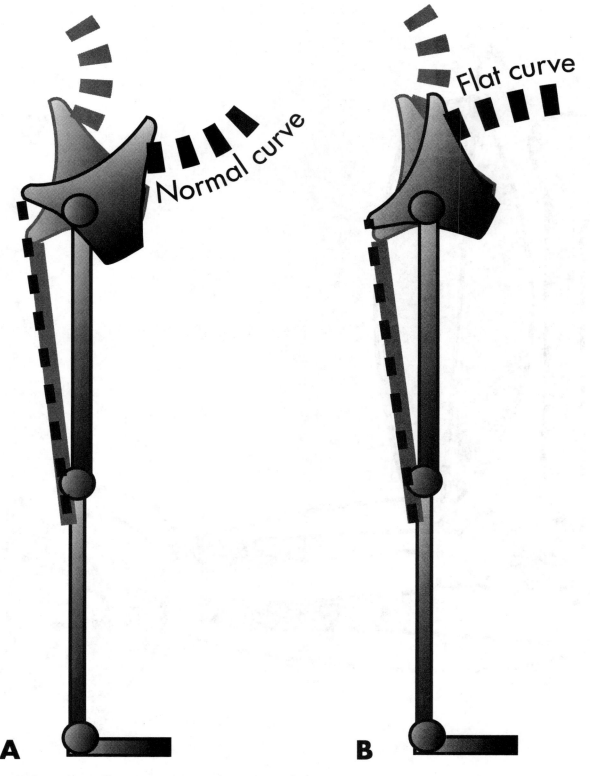

Normal curve

Flat curve

A

B

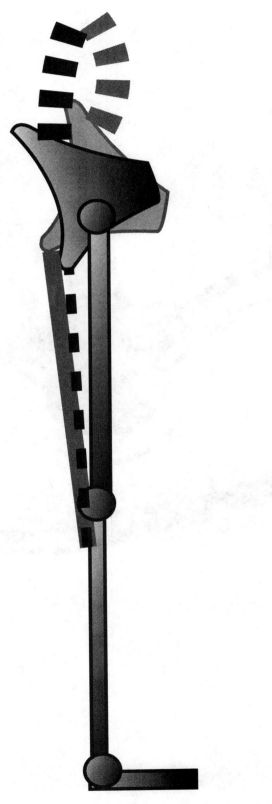

TM 36

Rotation of vertebral bodies in scoliosis (Figure 6-5)

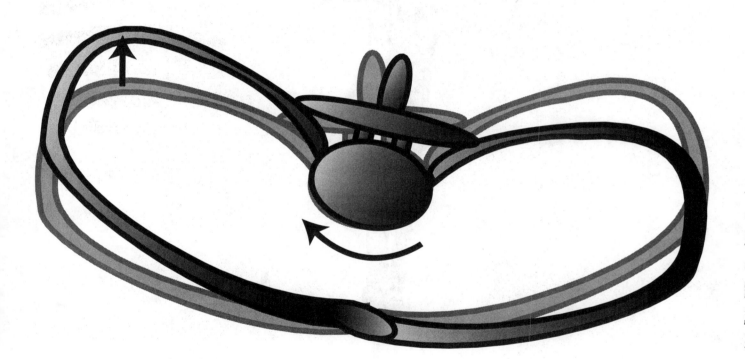

Erector spinae muscles in relation in vertebral axes (Figure 6-7)

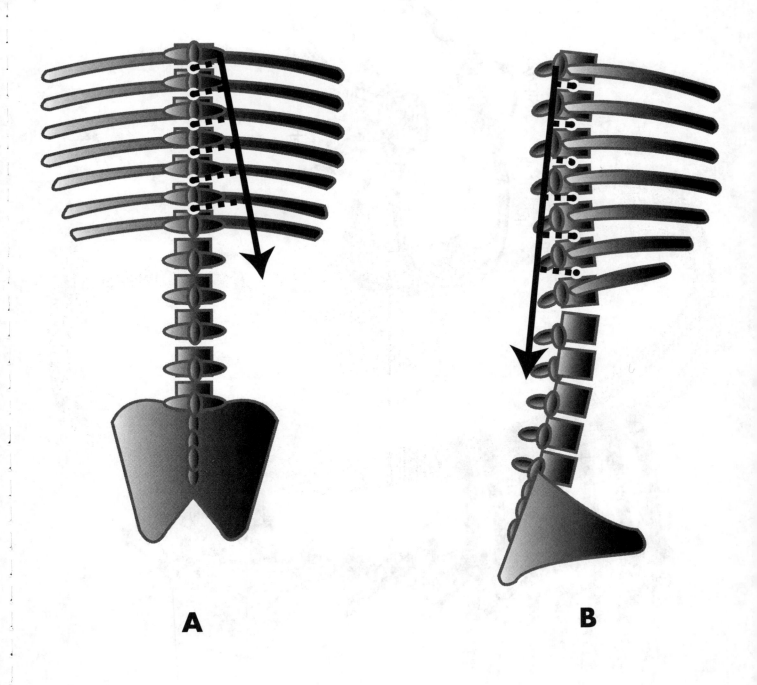

A

B

TM 38

Rotational effect of transversospinalis muscle (Figure 6-8)

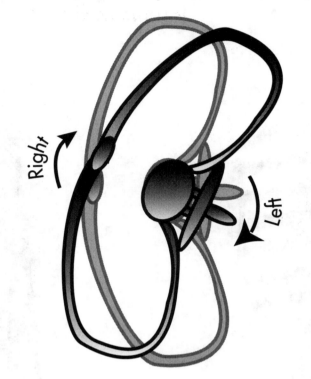

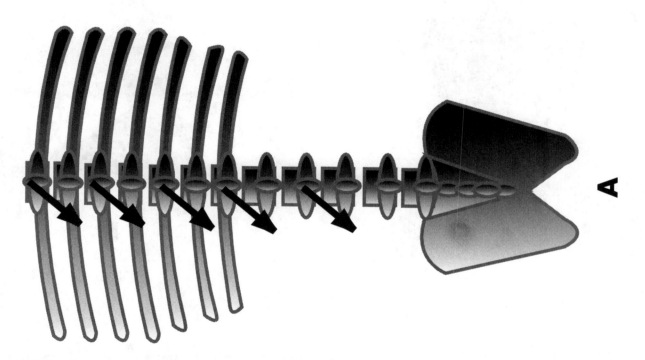

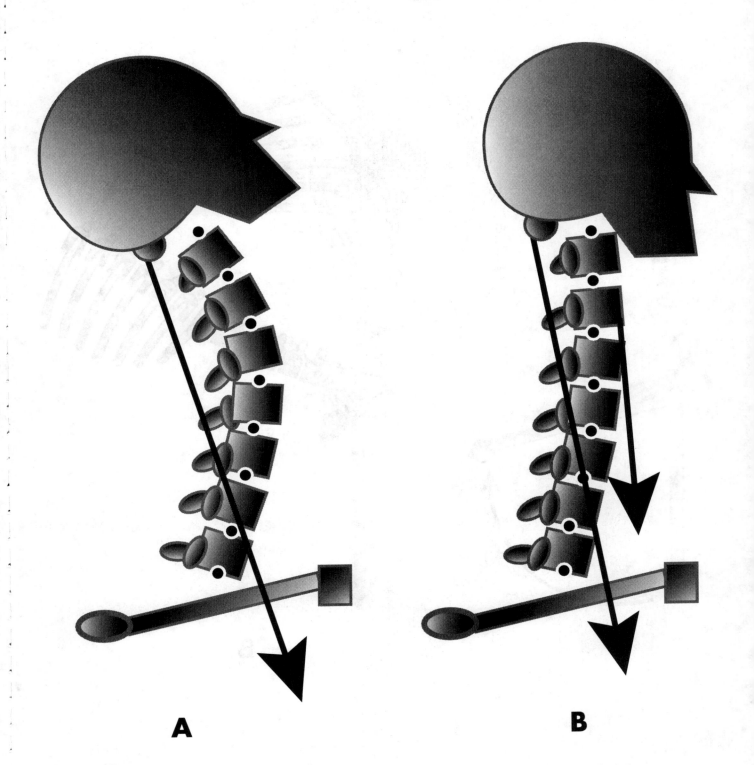

A

B

TM 40
Open- and closed-chain hip flexion (Figure 6-11)

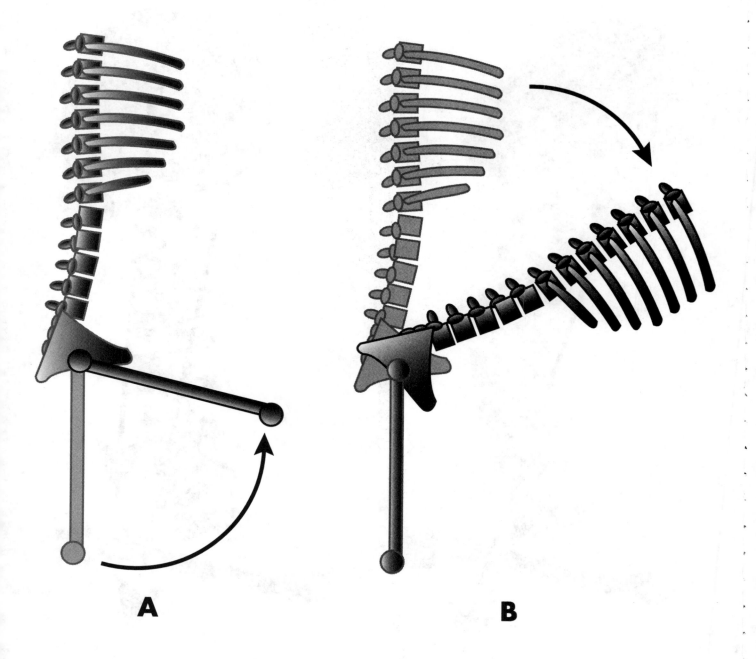

A

B

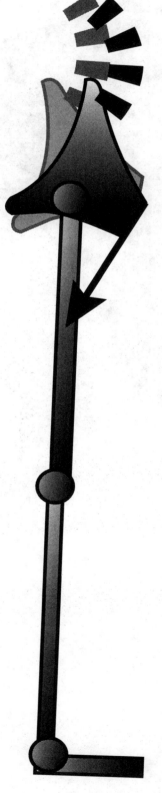

Greene/Roberts: Kinesiology: Movement in the Context of Activity
Copyright © 1999, Mosby, Inc.

TM 42
Arm abductors moving their origin (Figure 6-13)

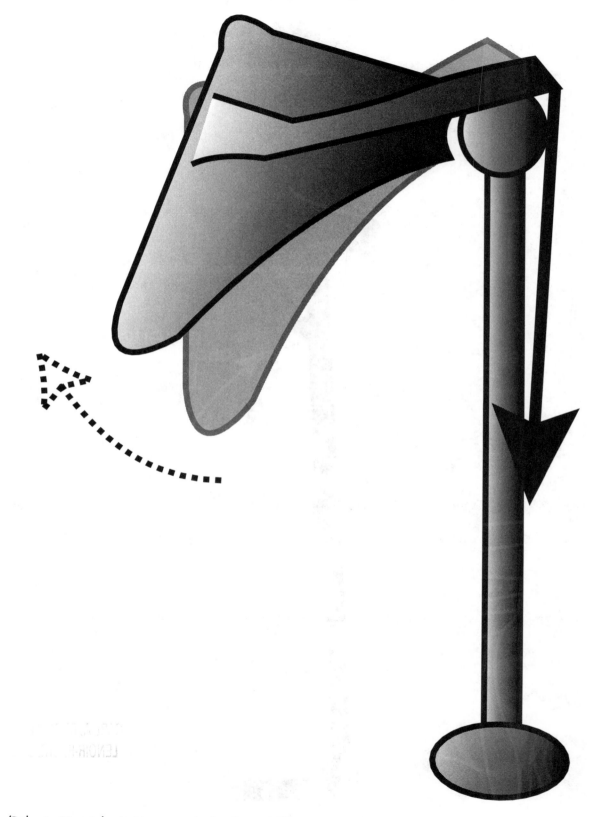

Erector spinae force when holding a 25-cm box (Figure 6-19)

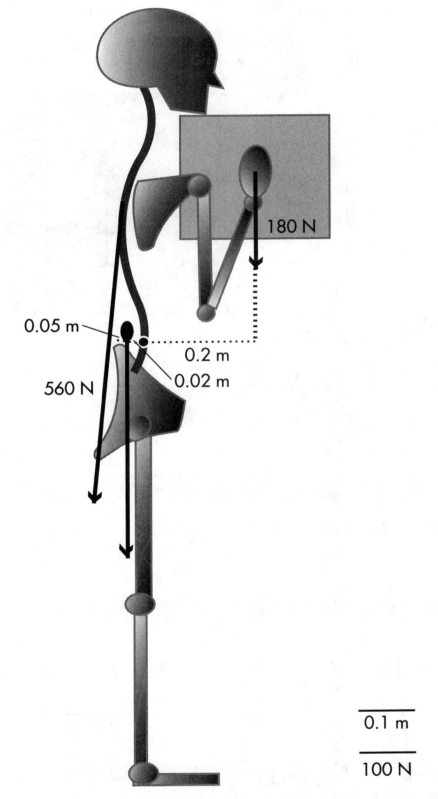

180 N

0.05 m

0.2 m

0.02 m

560 N

0.1 m

100 N

Greene/Roberts: Kinesiology: Movement in the Context of Activity

TM 44
Erector spinae force when holding a 46-cm box (Figure 6-20)

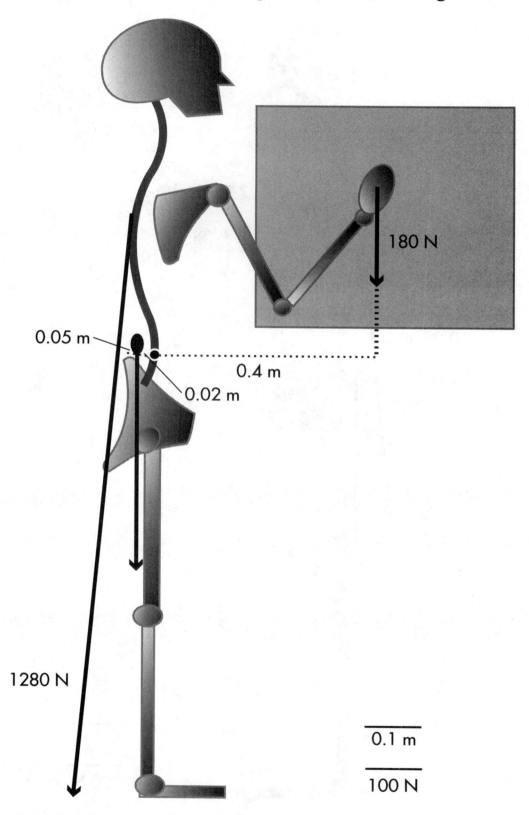

0.05 m

0.02 m

0.4 m

180 N

1280 N

0.1 m

100 N

Erector spinae force in standing (Figure 6-23)

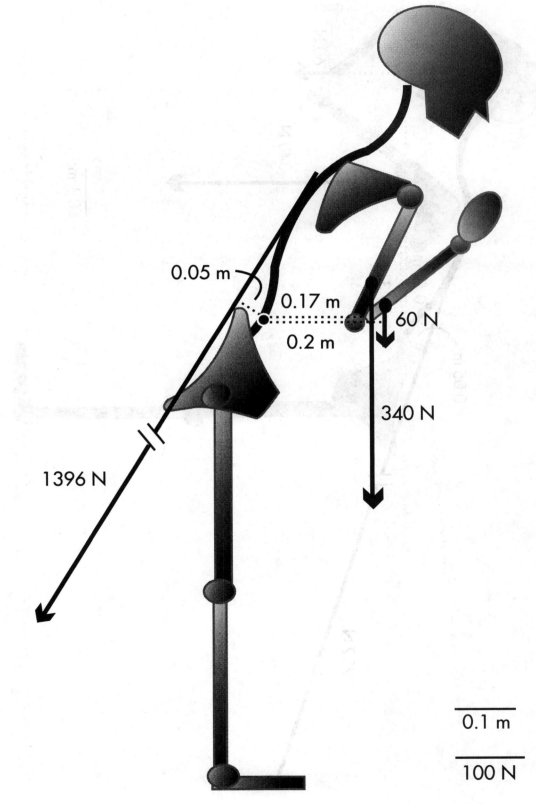

TM 46

Erector spinae force in forward bending (Figure 6-24)

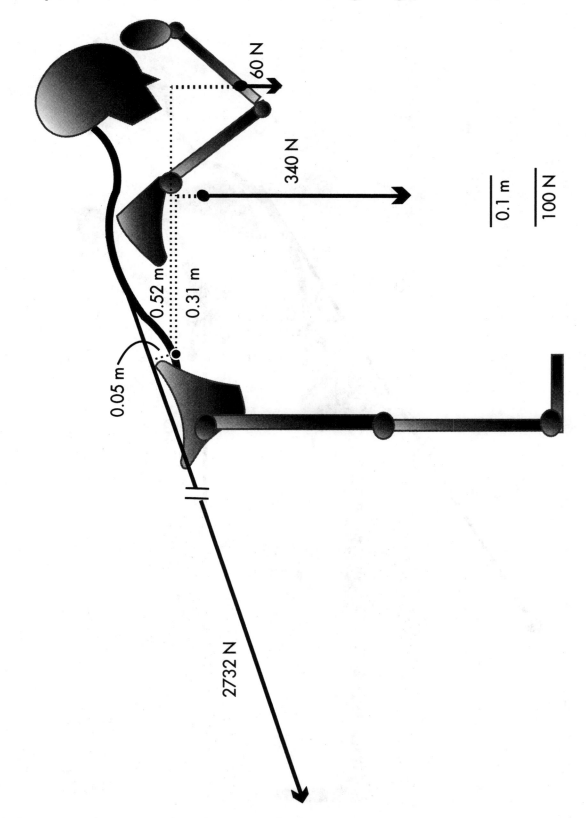

Scapular rotation likened to a steering wheel (Figure 7-2)

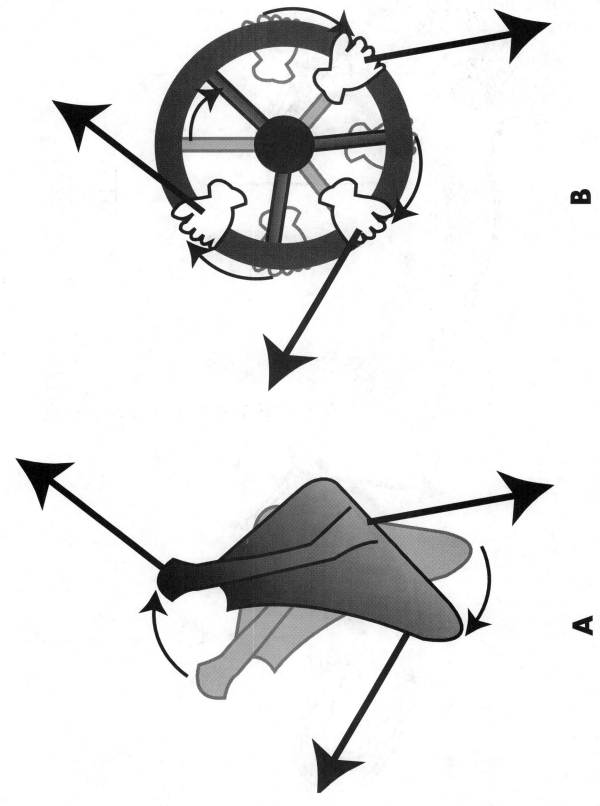

B

A

TM 48

Scapular winging due to a different attachment
of serratus anterior (Figure 7-3)

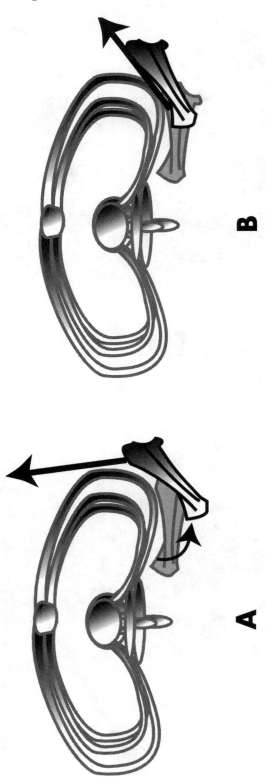

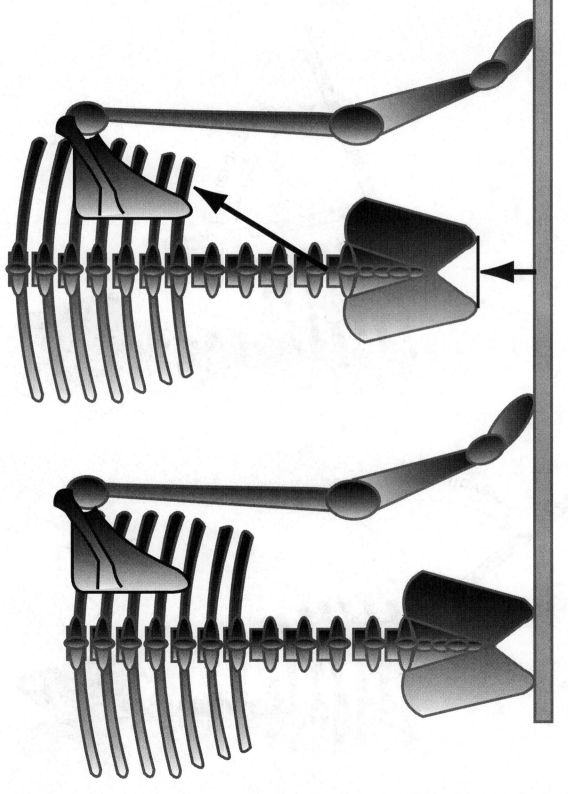

TM 50

Glenohumeral movement with and without
scapular stabilization (Figure 7-5)

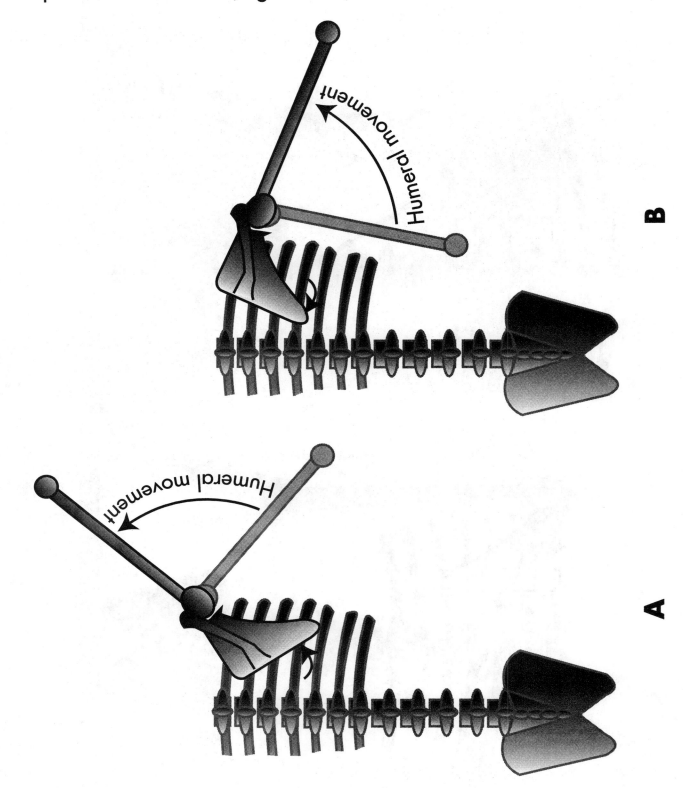

A

B

Downward pull of three rotator cuff muscles (Figure 7-6)

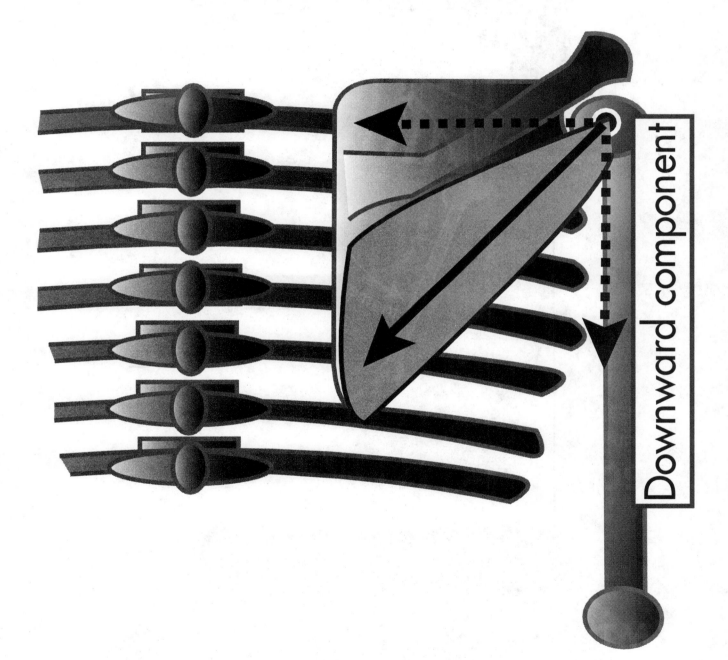

Downward component

Greene/Roberts: Kinesiology: Movement in the Context of Activity
Copyright © 1999, Mosby, Inc.

TM 52
Mechanism of glenohumeral subluxation (Figure 7-8)

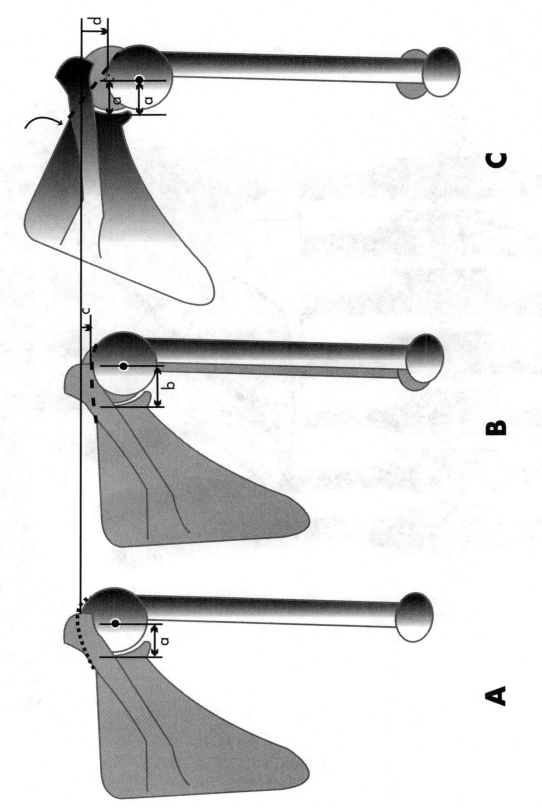

Changing the relationship of muscle pull (Figure 7-9)

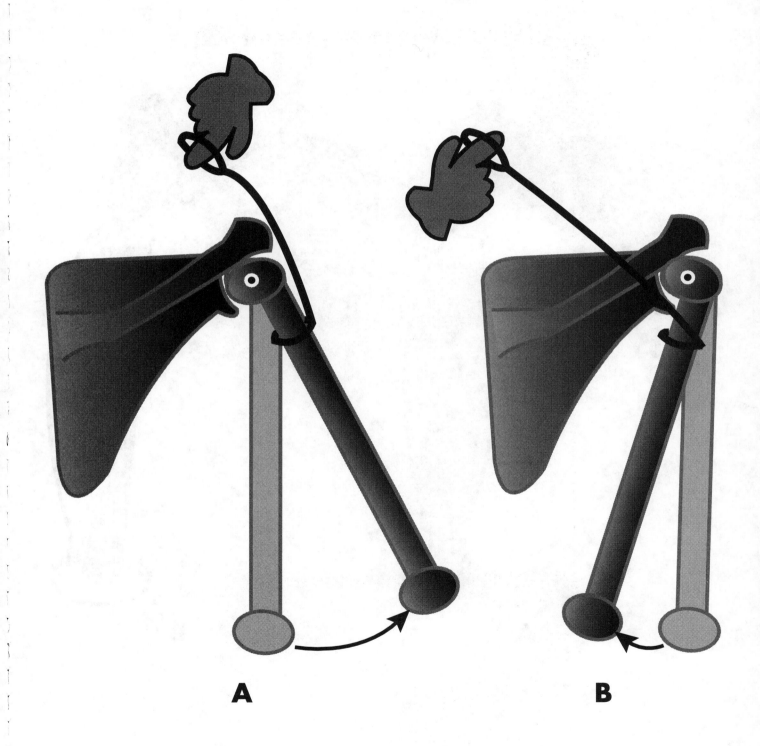

A

B

TM 54

Biceps as an abductor (Figure 7-10)

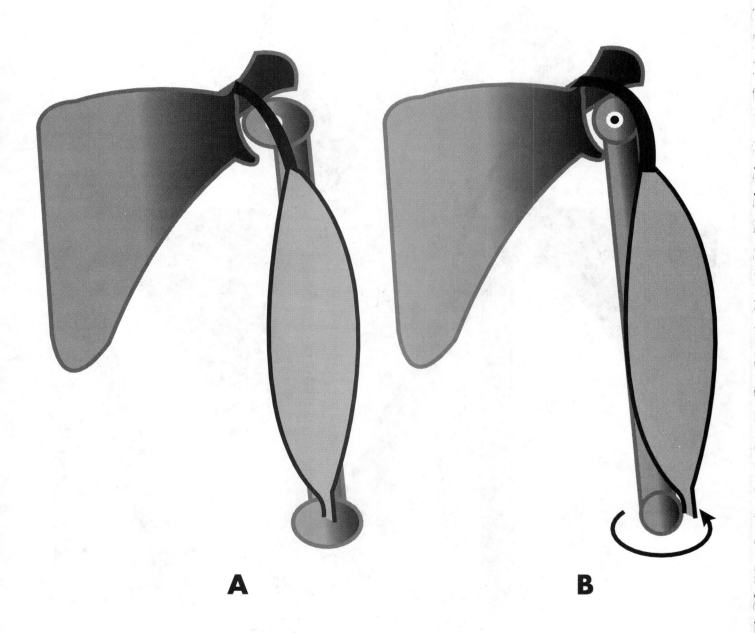

A

B

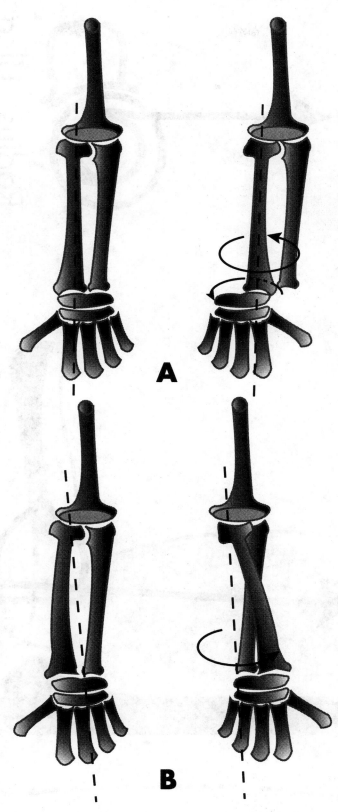

A

B

TM 56
Biceps spinning the radius like a top (Figure 7-12)

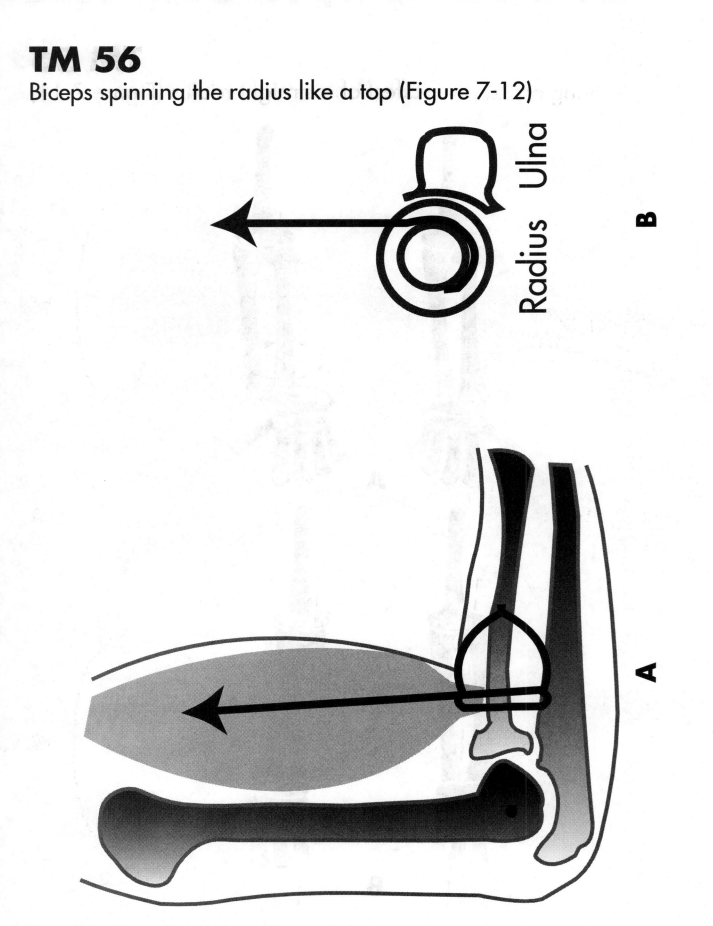

Radius   Ulna

B

A

Changing relationship of the brachioradialis (Figure 7-13)

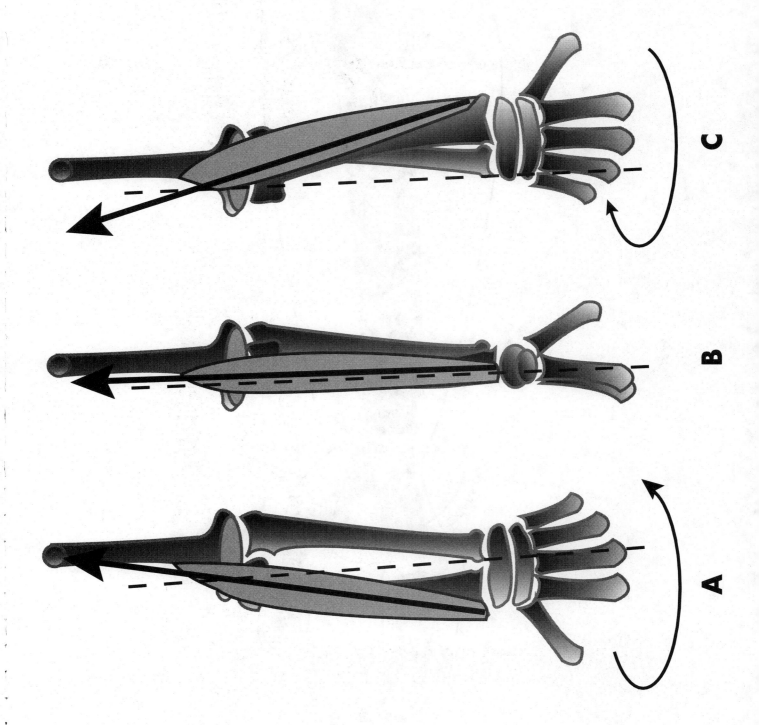

TM 58

Axes for wrist flexion and extension (Figure 8-1)

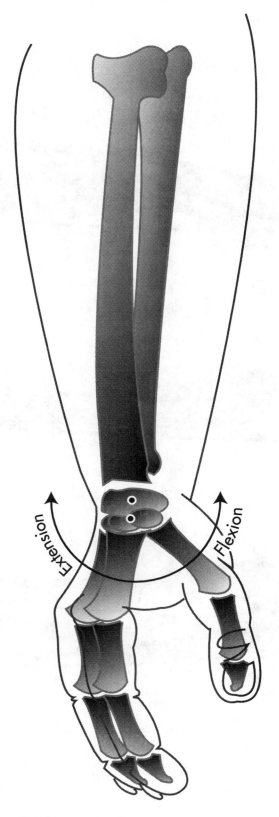

Extension

Flexion

Flexion, extension, and deviation moment arms for wrist muscles (Figure 8-2)

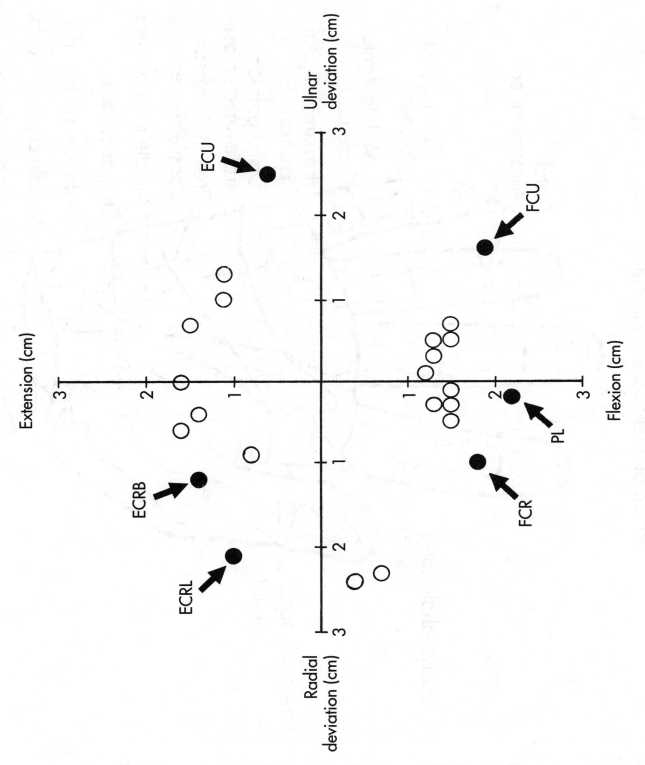

TM 60
Palmar skin creases overlying wrist and digital joints (Figure 8-3)

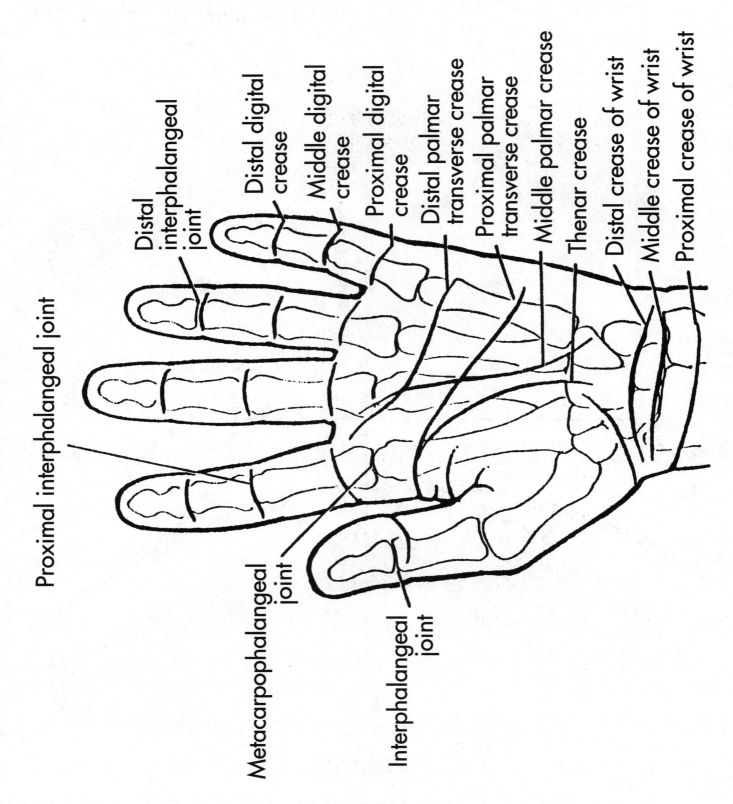

Distal interphalangeal joint

Distal digital crease

Middle digital crease

Proximal digital crease

Distal palmar transverse crease

Proximal palmar transverse crease

Middle palmar crease

Thenar crease

Distal crease of wrist

Middle crease of wrist

Proximal crease of wrist

Proximal interphalangeal joint

Metacarpophalangeal joint

Interphalangeal joint

A

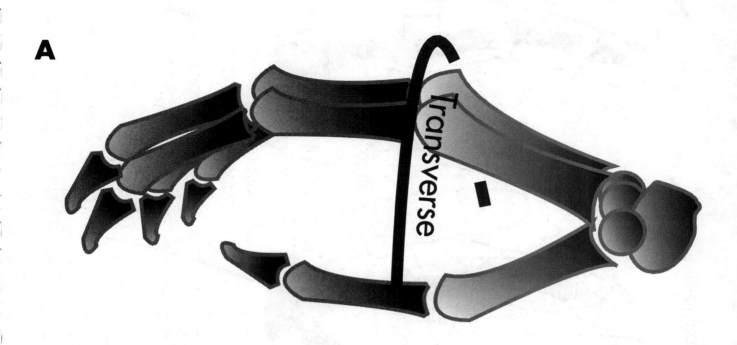

B

Longitudinal

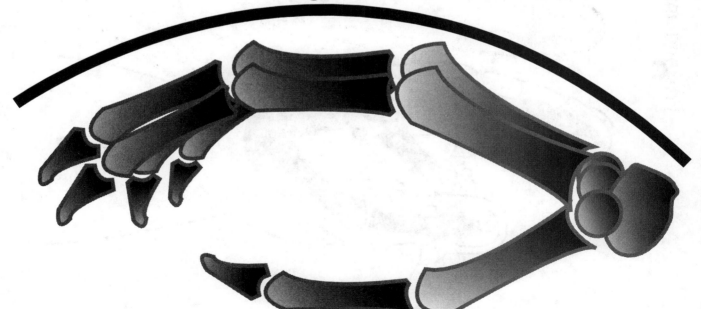

Greene/Roberts: Kinesiology: Movement in the Context of Activity
Copyright © 1999, Mosby, Inc.

TM 62

Relation of ligament length to joint position (Figure 8-5)

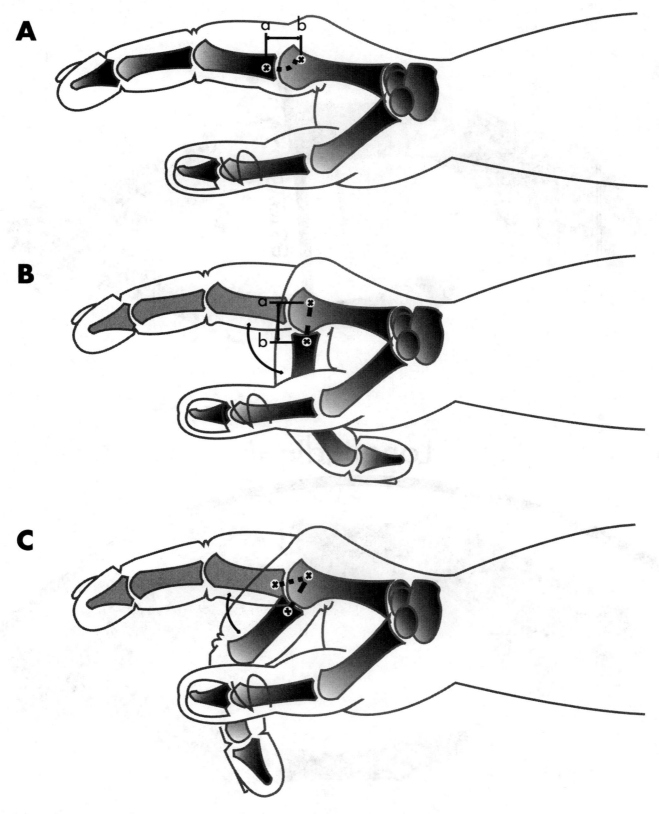

Wasting of finger flexor excursion at the wrist (Figure 8-8)

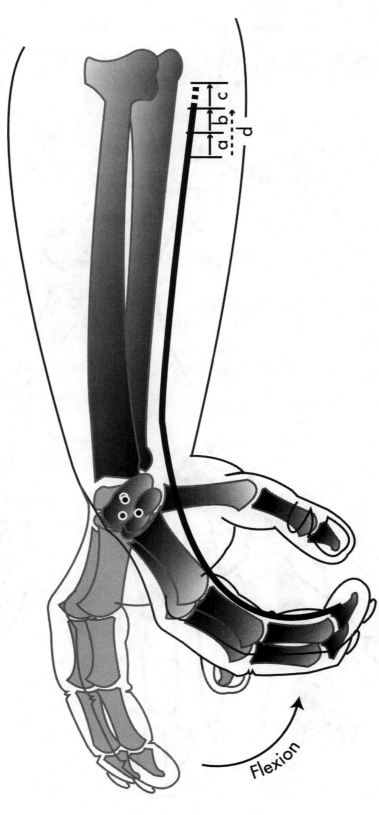

Flexion

TM 64
Intrinsic minus (Figure 8-10)

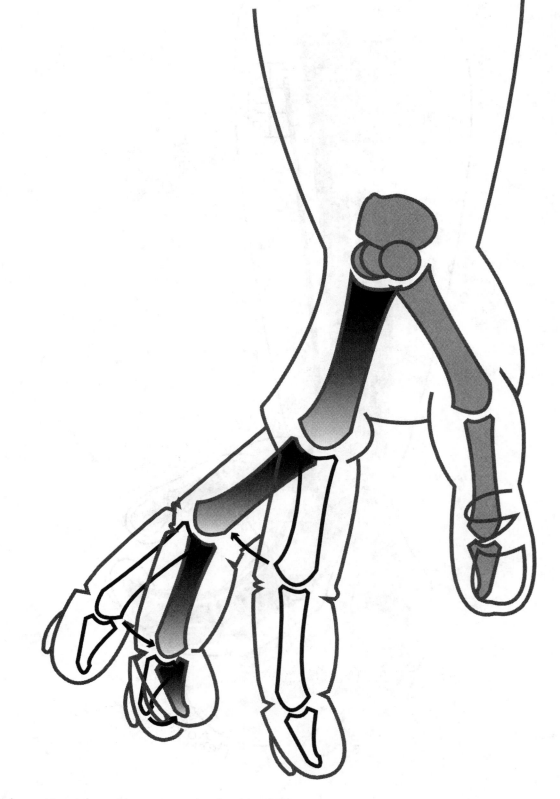

Extensor digitorum acting alone (Figure 8-11)

A

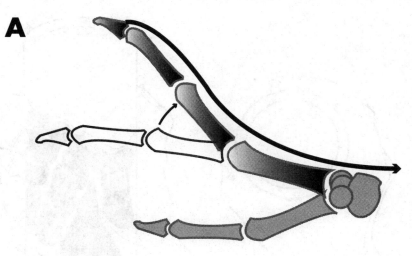

B

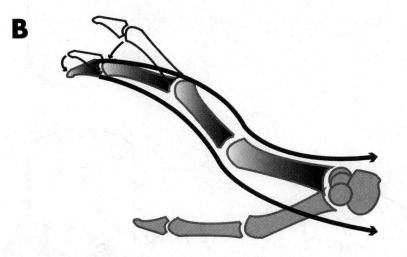

C

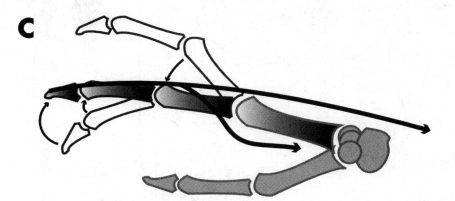

TM 66

Normal and intrinsic minus grasp (Figure 8-12)

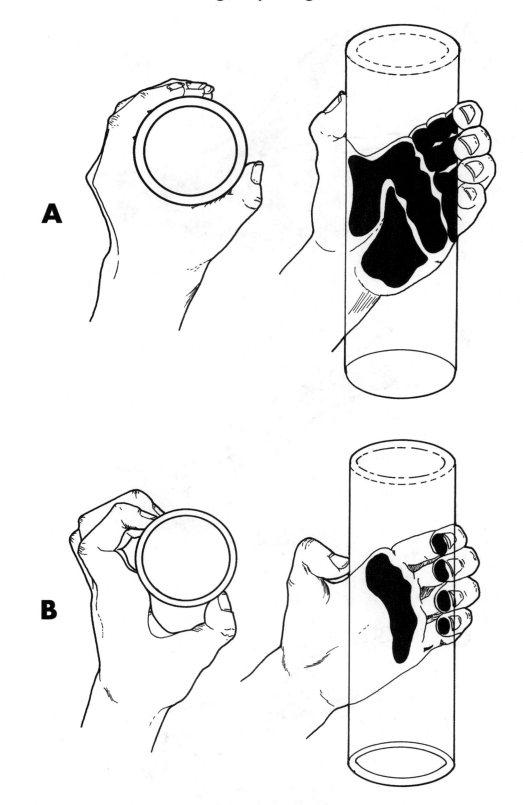

A

B

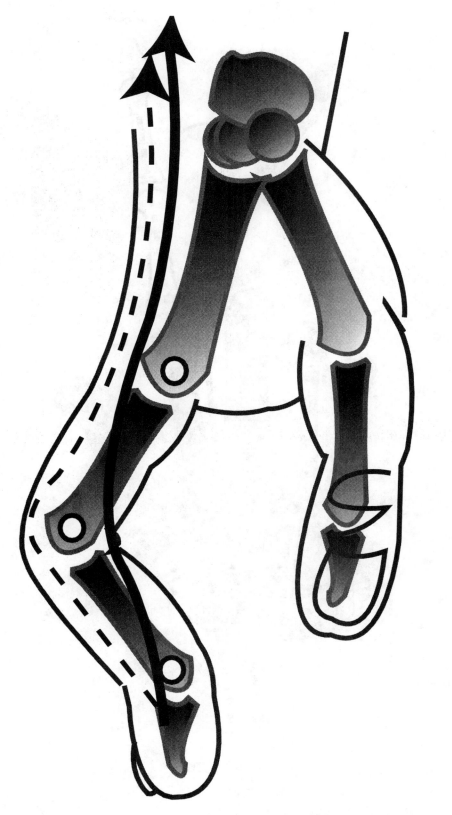

TM 68
Ulnar drift (Figure 8-14)

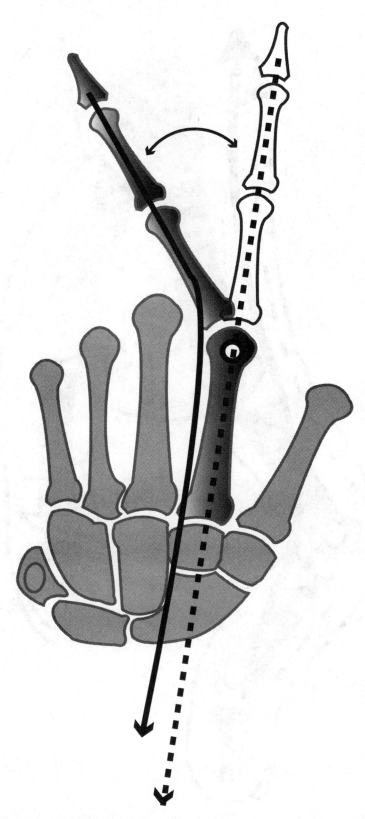

Tilting instead of gliding at the joint (Figure 8-15)

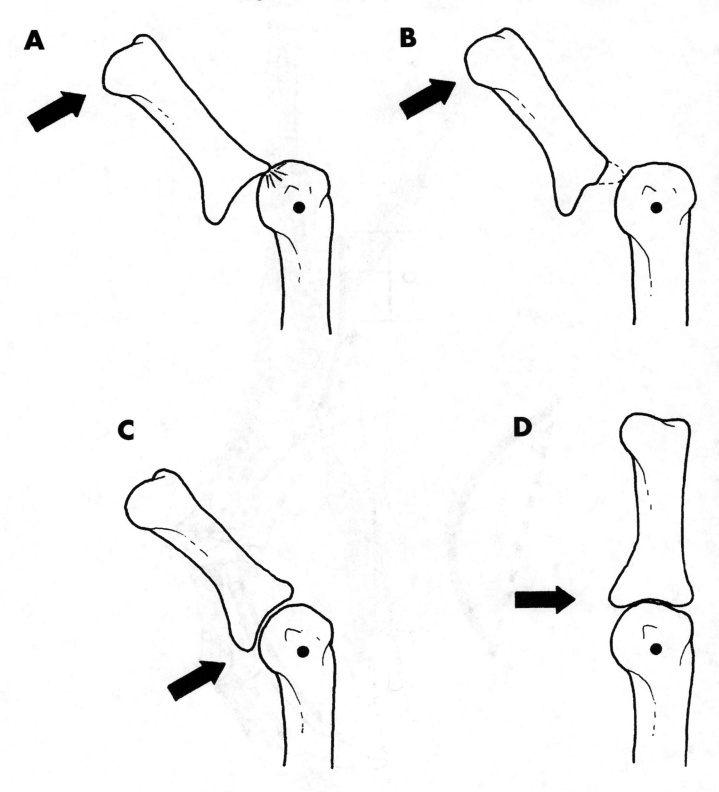

TM 70

Bowstringing (Figure 8-16)

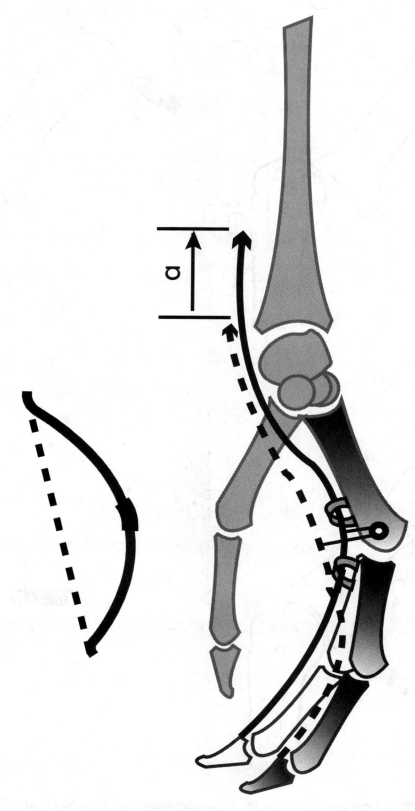

Excursion related to distance of insertion from axis of motion (Figure 8-17)

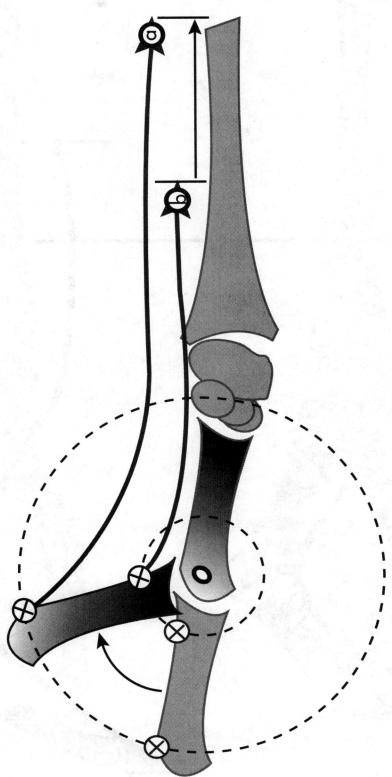

TM 72

Excursion and pulley damage (Figure 8-18)

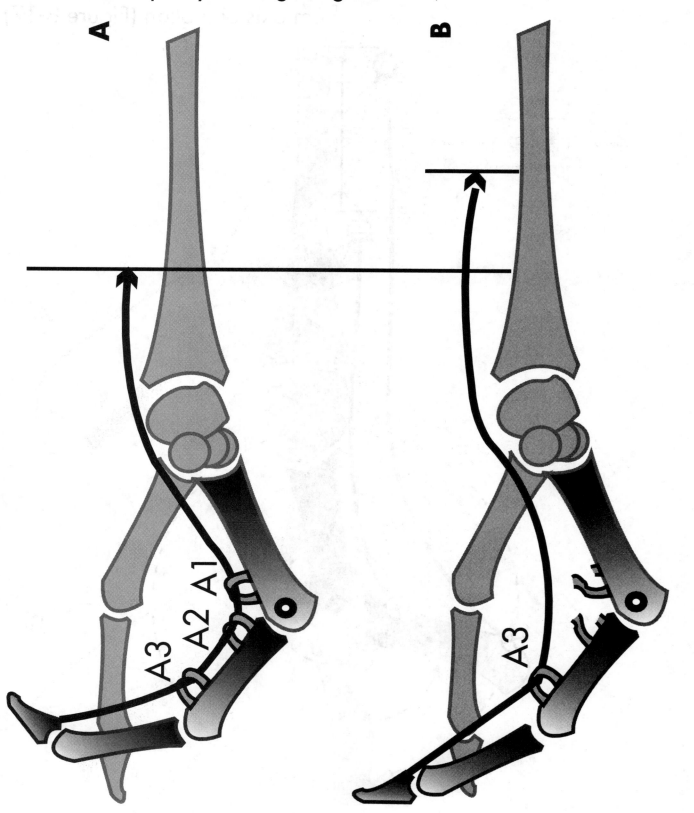

Torque range of motion (Figure 8-23)

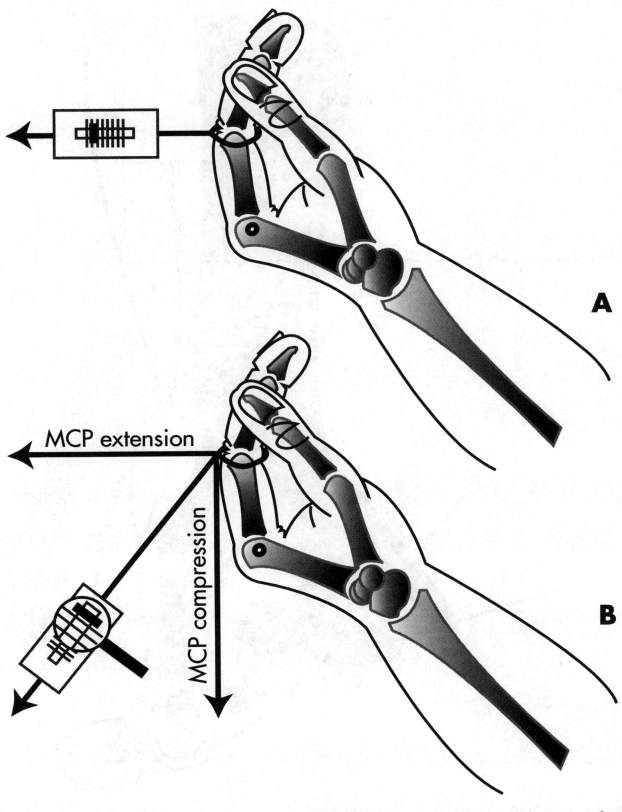

MCP extension

MCP compression

A

B

TM 74
Angle of pull in splinting (Figure 8-24)

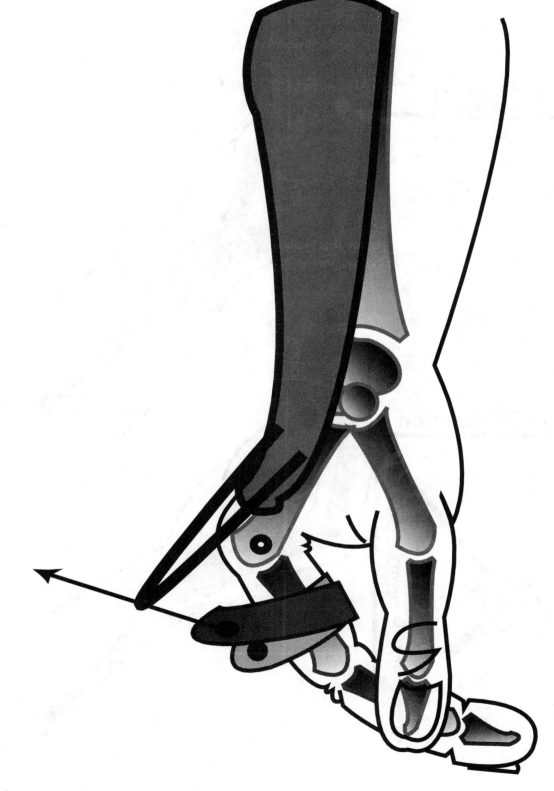

Grasp type affecting force requirements (Figure 8-27)

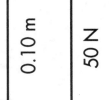

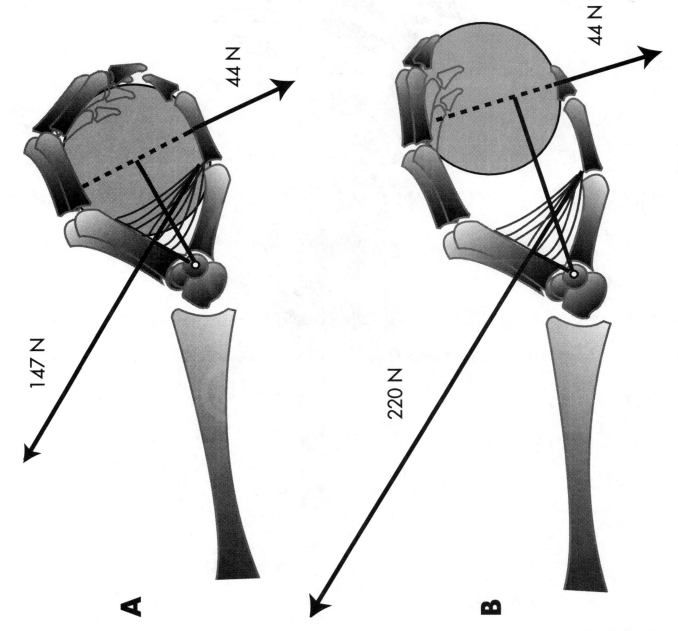

TM 76

Posture at the hip with weak or absent hip flexors (Figure 9-1)

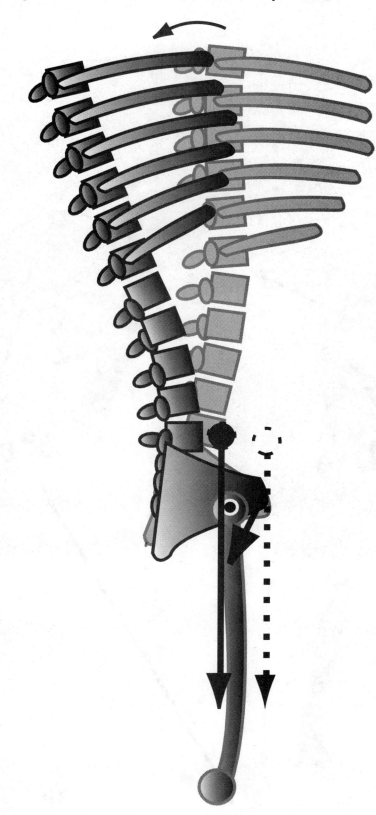

Gravity's abduction moment at the hip (Figure 9-2)

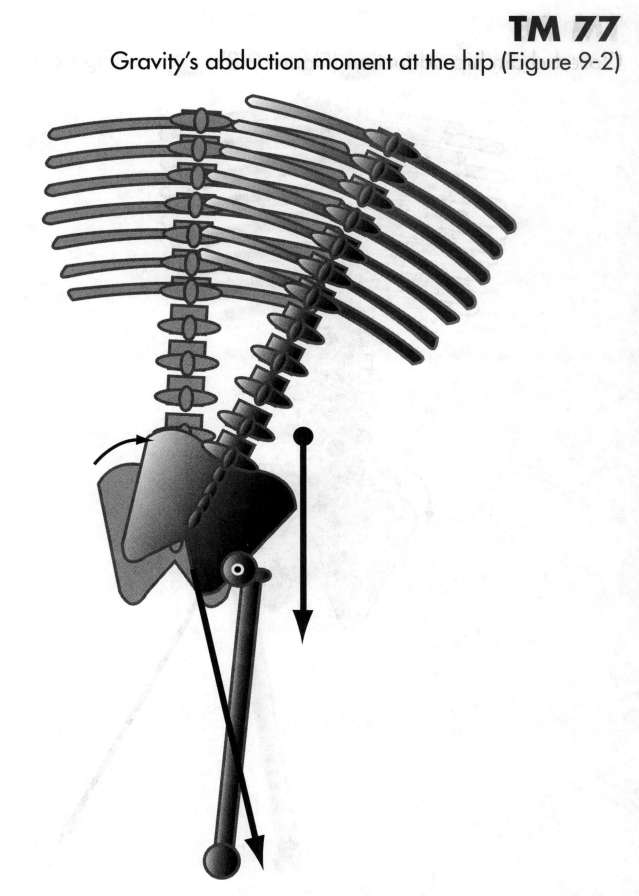

TM 78

Closed-chain hip adduction (Figure 9-3)

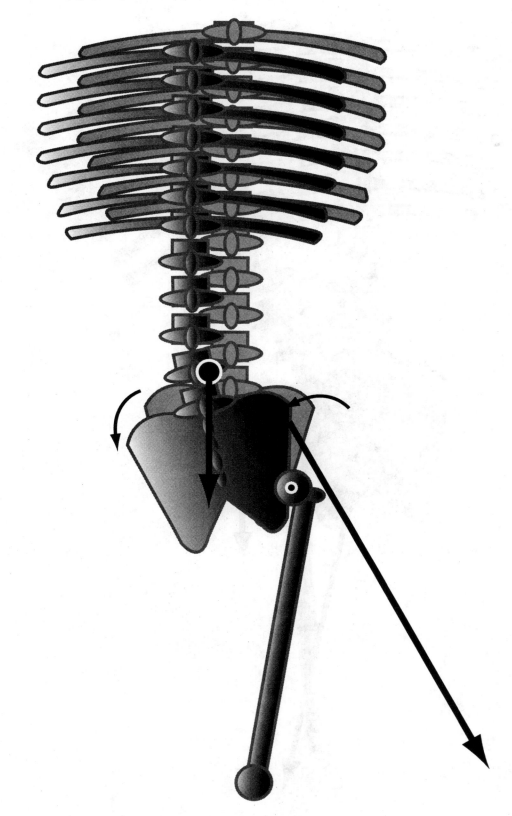

Open- and closed-chain dorsiflexion (Figure 9-5)

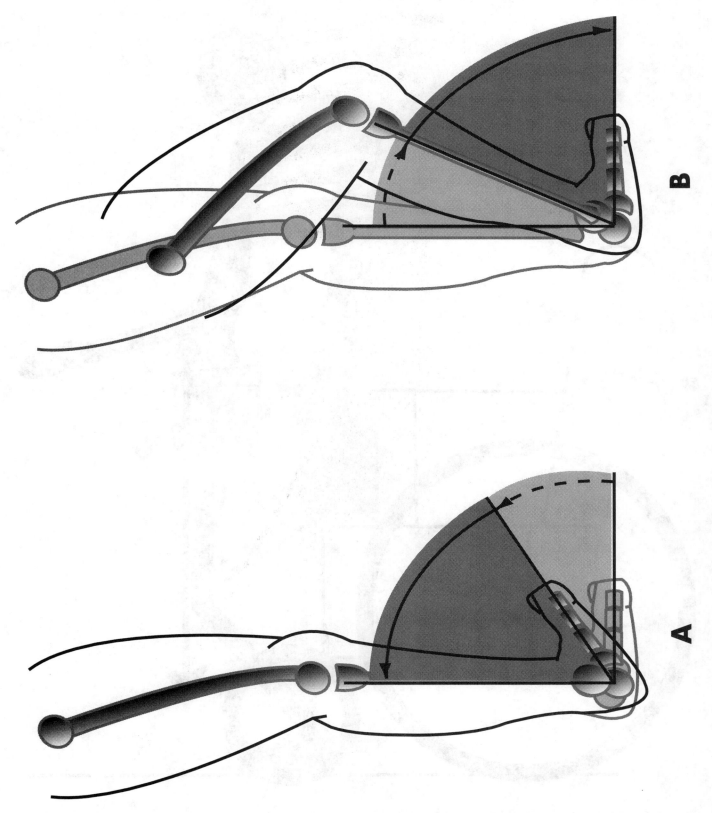

B

A

A too-close transitional base of support (Figure 9-8)

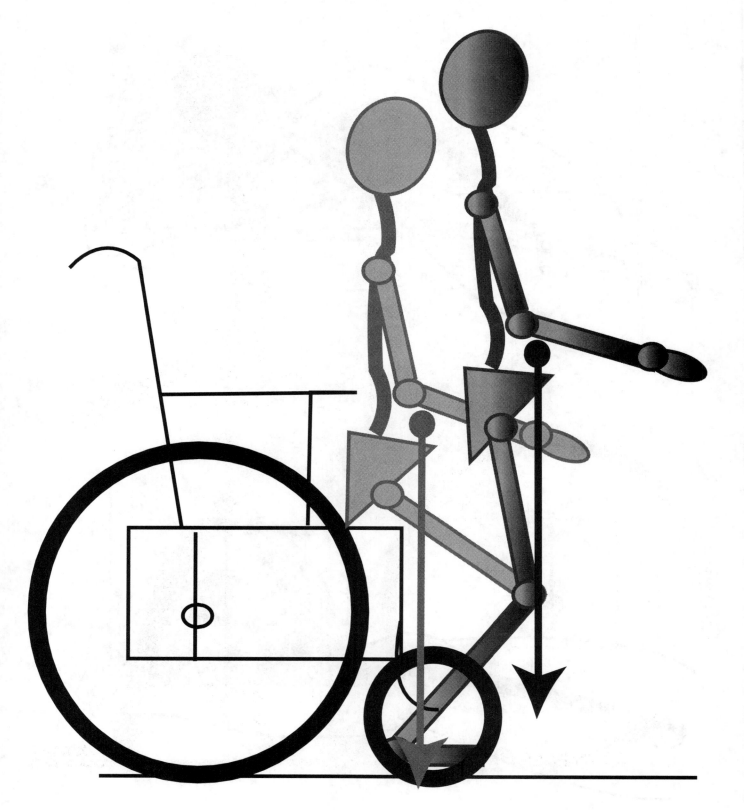

A too-far transitional base of support (Figure 9-9)

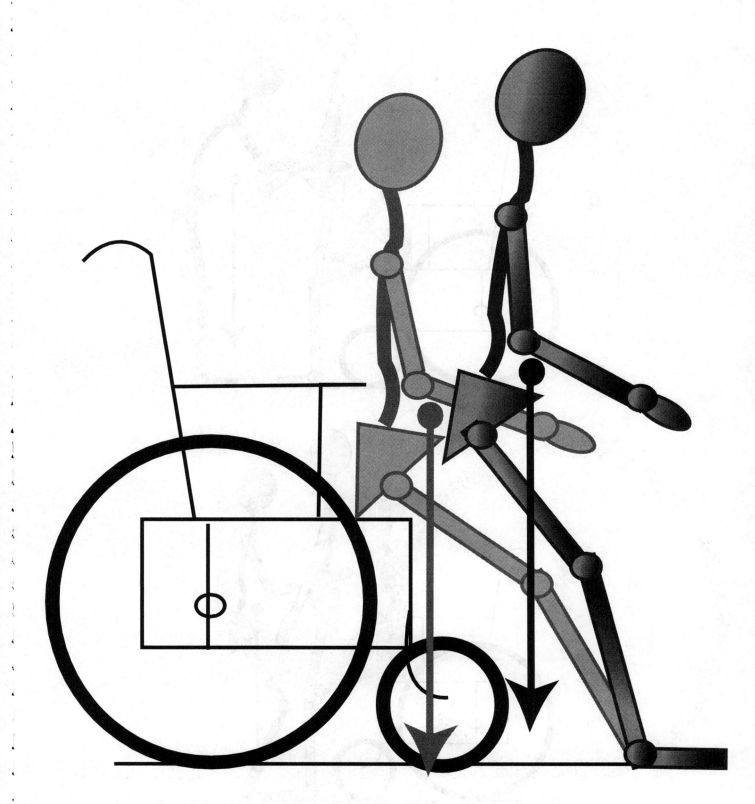

TM 82

Practitioner's center of gravity in transfers (Figure 9-10)

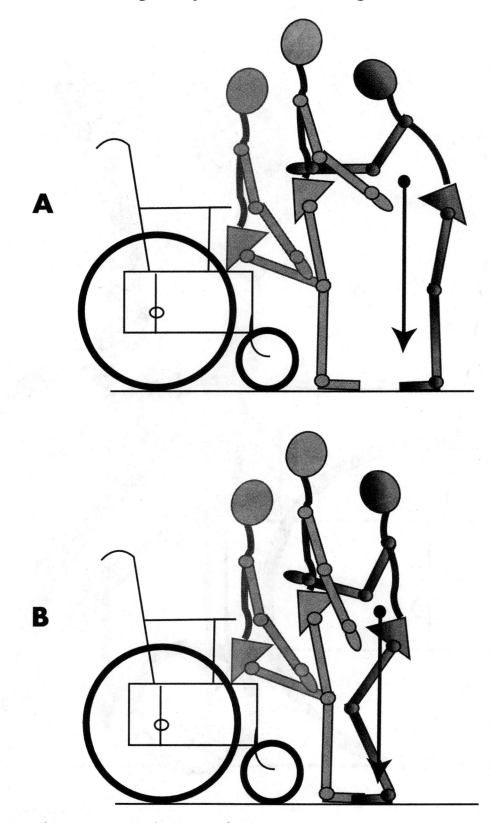

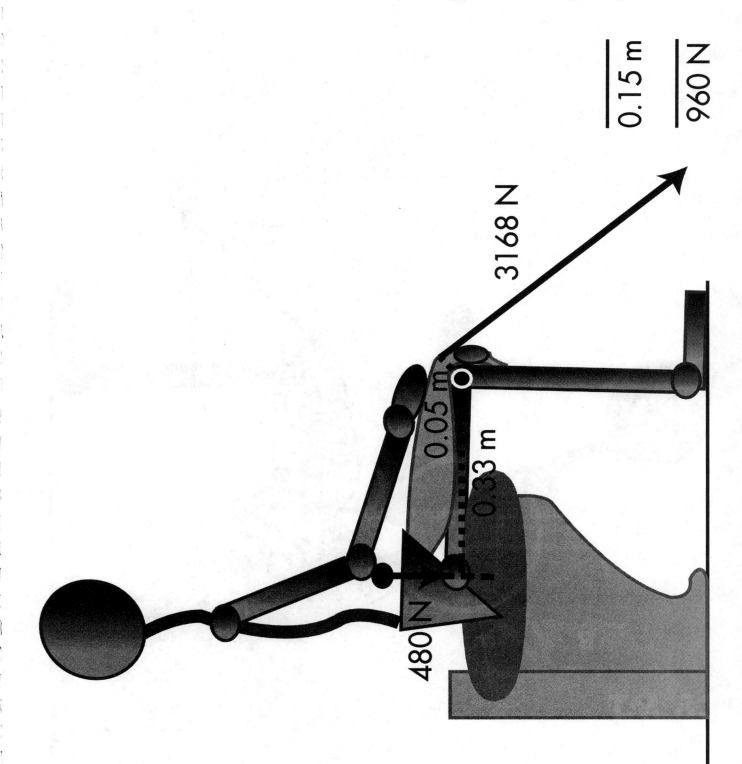

0.15 m

960 N

3168 N

0.05 m

0.33 m

480 N

TM 84
Standing from forward leaning (Figure 9-14)

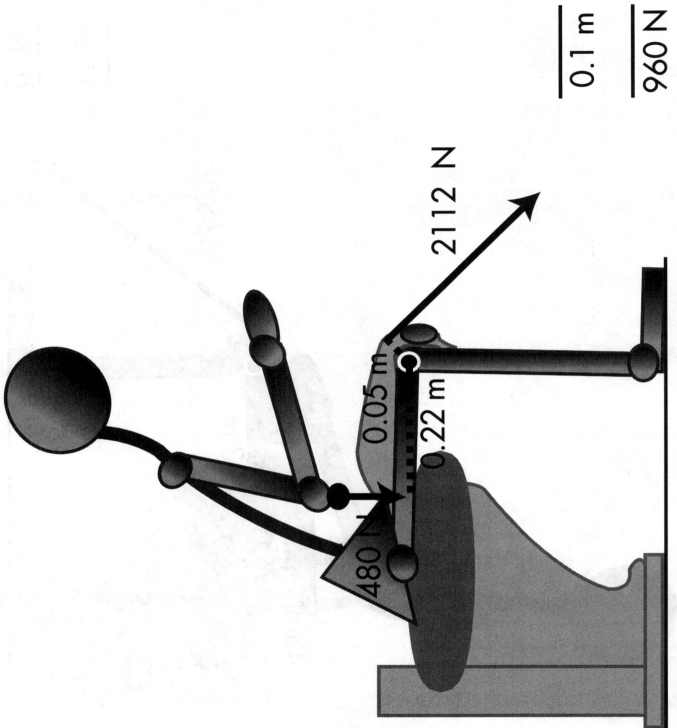

2112 N

0.1 m

960 N

0.05 m

0.22 m

480 N

Semi recliner and the projected center of gravity (Figure 9-16)

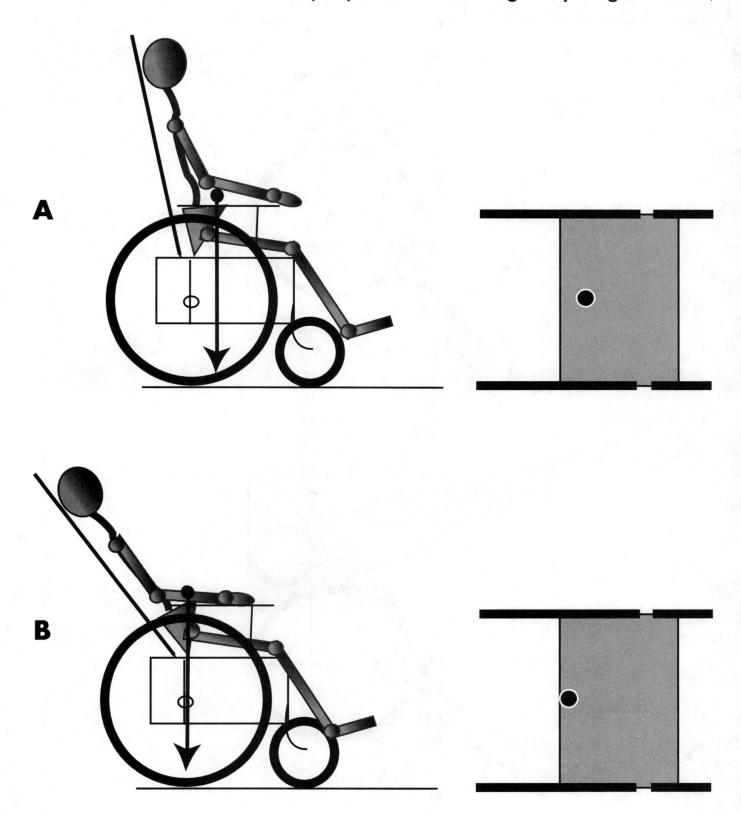

TM 86

Instability of a quick start with the wheelchair
back reclined (Figure 9-17)

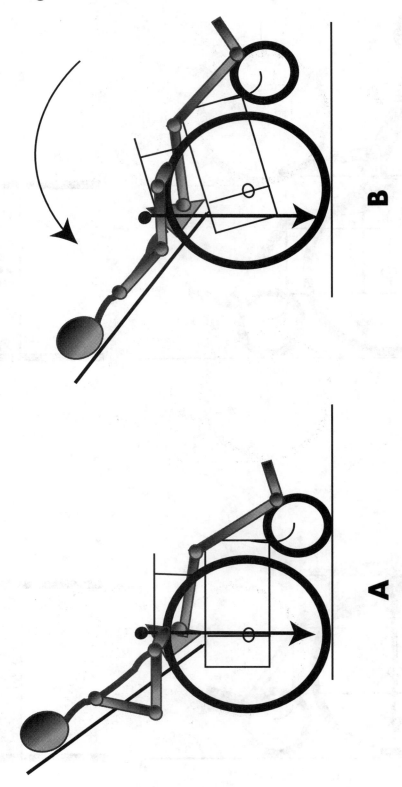

Casters and base of support (Figure 9-20)

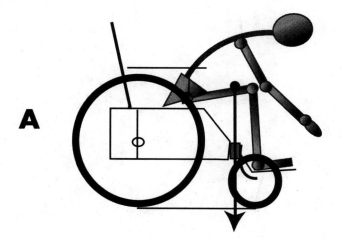

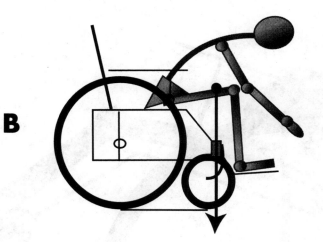

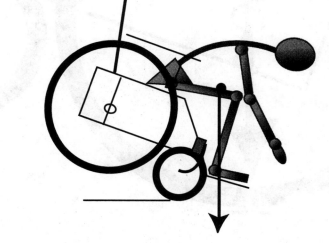

TM 88

Balance in a "wheelie" (Figure 9-21)

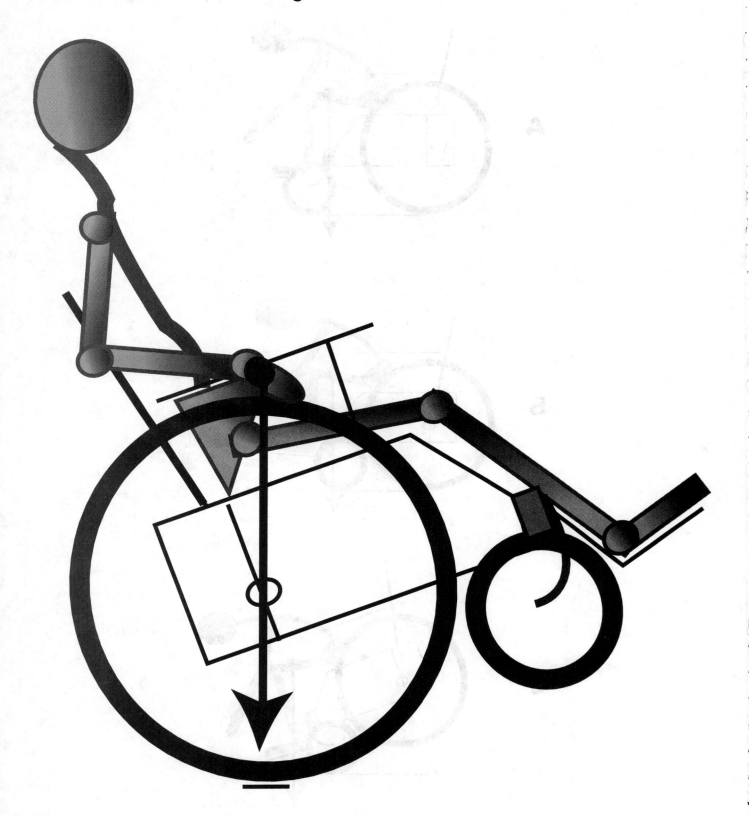

Camber and base of support (Figure 9-22)

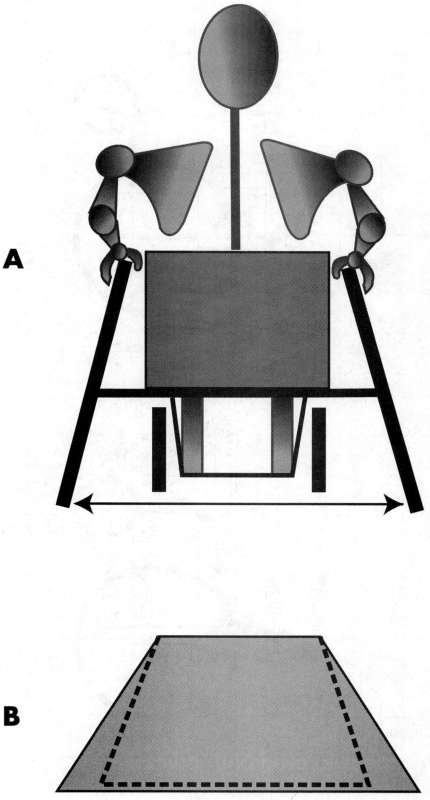

A

B

TM 90

Shift in center of gravity following amputation (Figure 9-23)

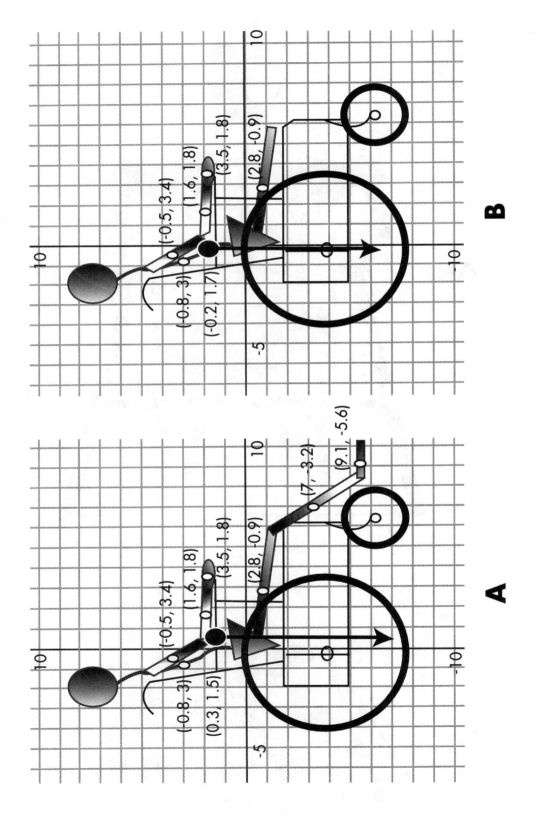